Master's Guide for the
Emergency Medicine
Sub-Internship

Daniel G. Ostermayer, MD

Welcome

Master's Guide for the EM Sub-I provides an advanced set of pearls that will quickly augment your emergency medicine knowledge. The chapters, organized by system, serve as a way to jumpstart your career in Emergency Medicine and take your knowledge to the next level. I recommend pairing each chapter with a corresponding core emergency medicine textbook chapter for maximal educational benefit.

Cardiovascular

STEMI

- Complete coronary artery occlusion Full-thickness transmural infarction
- ≥1 mm (0.1 mV) ST segment elevation in limb leads
- ≥ 2 mm ST segment elevation in precordial leads
- Findings present in at least 2 anatomically contiguous leads

Treatment

- Oxygen only if saturations are <95%
- Chewed aspirin 324mg
- Nitroglycerin for pain relief
- Heparin (anticoagulation for cardiac catheterization)\
- Additional platelet inhibition (clopidogrel, ticagrelor)
- Acute percutaneous intervention or thrombolytics
- Goal for PCI is EMS to cath. lab in less than 90 minutes

Fourth Universal Definition of STEMI

- 1 mm of ST elevation in any two contiguous leads except V2 and V3. or
- In women: 1.5mm elevation in V2 and V3
- In men under 40: 2.5mm elevation in V2 and V3
- In men 40 and older: 2mm elevation in V2 and V3

NSTEMI

- Incomplete coronary artery occlusion
- ST depressions and T wave inversions

STABLE ANGINA

- Flow limiting plaque causes cardiac pain with exertion

UNSTABLE ANGINA

- Flow limiting plaque causes pain at rest but can quickly escalate to an acute occlusion

PARTIAL CORONARY OCCLUSION

- Presents as unstable or stable angina or with a new Left Bundle Branch Block, Wellens' Syndrome, or De Winter's T-waves

WELLENS' SYNDROME

- A history of cardiac related chest but the patient at the time of the abnormal ECG may be pain free
- Deeply inverted or biphasic T waves in V2-3, (highly specific for a critical stenosis of the left anterior descending artery)

DE WINTER'S T-WAVES

- ST depression and peaked T-waves in the precordial leads.
- "HyperK" looking T wave

NEW LEFT BUNDLE BRANCH BLOCK

- If in the setting of chest pain then assume acute coronary occlusion

Sgarbossa criteria can help differentiate STEMI from LBBB

- **≥3 points = 98% probability of STEMI**
    - ST elevation ≥1 mm in a lead with upward QRS complex (concordant) - 5 points
    - ST depression ≥1 mm in lead V1, V2, or V3 - 3 points
    - ST elevation ≥5 mm in a lead with downward QRS complex (discordant) - 2 points
- **Smith's modification**
    - Changes the 3rd rule of original Sgarbossa's Criteria to be ST depression OR elevation discordant with the QRS complex and with a magnitude of at least 25% of the QRS
- These criteria are specific, but not sensitive for myocardial infarction. Point total ≥ 3 is reported to have a specificity of 90% for diagnosing myocardial infarction.

STEMI MIMICS

- **LV aneurysm** (often from prior MI)
- **Benign Early Repolarization** (often concave large T-waves in V2-V3)
- **Left Ventricular Hypertrophy**
    - Can have ST depression and T-wave inversions in V5-5V6
    - Elevation in V1-2
- **Coronary spasm (prinzmetal's angina)**
- **Myocarditis (usually diffuse in all leads without anatomic distribution)**
- **Pericarditis**
    - ST elevation in all leads except aVR and V1
    - PR depressions in all leads
- **Hyperkalemia**

ANTERIOR MI

- Location: Left anterior Descending artery (LAD)
- Left Ventricle involved with a large portion of myocardial tissue
- Prognosis is poor if not emergently revascularized
- May cause high degree heart block due to infarct of the conduction
- ST elevation in V1 - V4 with reciprocal depressions (III, avF)
- Can progress rapidly to acute cardiogenic shock
- Complications can involve:
    - Acute arrhythmias (VT, VF)
    - LV Aneurysm (often 2-4 weeks post MI)

INFERIOR MI

- The inferior portion of the myocardium **partially extends posteriorly (RV)**
- An inferior MI can be an isolated inferior MI or an **inferior MI** with **RV extension (25% of patients)**
- ST segment elevation in II, III, avF
- RCA lesion
- Complications can include
    - Bradycardia (from a vagal response)
    - 2nd degree AV block - types I and II (requires pacing)

INFERIOR MI WITH RV EXTENSION

- 25% of interior infarcts
- ST segment elevation in II, III, aVF
- If there is ST elevation in V1 or in lead III > lead II then there should be concern for RV extension
- Perform a right sided ECG lead to help diagnose RV extension
- 1 mm ST elevation in RV4 or RV3
- RV extension inferior MI is preload dependent
  - Caution with nitrates which decrease preload
- If not no signs of pulmonary edema then patients should be given a fluid bolus (500mL)

LATERAL MI

- Lesion in circumflex
- ST elevations in I, aVL, V5, V6
- Reciprocal changes in II, III, aVF

POSTERIOR MI

- Infarct of the RCA or circumflex artery
- Due to the anterior arrangement of the ECG a posterior MI often doesn't present with a STEMI
- ST depression in V1, V2, V3
- A posterior ECG can reveal the "hidden" ST elevations
- ST elevations in the posterior V7,V8, and V9 leads

PCI COMPLICATIONS:

- Ventricular wall or Mitral valve rupture
  - Can present with flash pulmonary edema with new murmur
- Left free wall rupture (shows a new large pleural effusion)

AORTIC ANEURYSM

- The majority of abdominal aneurysms are infrarenal
- During acute rupture the SBP target is 100 mmHg

Risk Factors include

- Smoking
- Atherosclerosis
- HTN
- Age >65
- Marfan's Syndrome

Diagnostic findings

- Acute bruit
- Pulsatile abdominal mass
- Absent distant pulses
- Abdominal ultrasound can visually confirm

AORTIC DISSECTION

Presentation

- Extremely hypertensive patient with ripping/tearing chest pain radiating to the back
- Also can have neurologic deficits such as bilateral lower extremity paralysis
- A proximal aortic dissection can present with a regurgitation murmur if dissection extends to the aortic root (diastolic murmur)
- **Type A - Involves any portion of ascending aorta**
- **Type B - Isolated to descending aorta**

Treatment

- Decrease shear forces on dissecting flap by using Esmolol to achieve a goal HR < 60.
- Esmolol - advantage of short half life, easily titratable
- Bolus 0.1-0.5mg/kg over 1min; infuse 0.025-0.2mg/kg/min
- Add vasodilators once HR is < 60 (nicardipine or nitroprusside)

MYXOMA

- Benign cardiac tumor often presenting with an "atrial plop"

- Can cause intermittent atrial outflow obstruction leading to syncope/cardiac arrest
- Requires surgical resection

ACUTE AORTIC REGURGITATION

- Diastolic murmur
- If dissection related there can be tearing chest pain
- May have an MI on ECG and a pericardial effusion

ACUTE MITRAL REGURGITATION

- Can present with acute pulmonary edema or acute syncope
- Pan-systolic murmur

AORTIC STENOSIS

- Generally a chronic disease with an acute presentation once severe
- Patients can present with acute congestive heart failure, arrhythmia, angina, or syncope
- A systolic murmur that radiates to the carotid with a delated carotid upstroke
- Patients are Preload dependent due to flow limiting stenosis.
  - Extreme sensitivity to vasodilators such as nitrates

DEEP VEIN THROMBOSIS AND THROMBOEMBOLISM

- **Imaging gold standards:**
  - Ultrasound for DVT
  - CTA for PE

Phlegmasia alba dolens (milk leg)

- Swollen and white leg because of early compromise of arterial flow secondary from extensive DVT
- Requires thrombolytic therapy

Phlegmasia cerulea dolens (blue leg)

- More advanced and considered a precursor of frank venous gangrene

• Requires thrombolytic therapy

Calf DVT

• If no other proximal DVTS then the calf DVT can be treated with outpatient follow-up with serial ultrasounds without anticoagulation
• **All DVTs should receive LMWH (safe in pregnancy)**
• **Decreased dosing of LMWH if in renal failure due to renal clearance.**

VENTRICULAR ANEURYSM

• Can occur weeks after an transmural myocardial infarction
• Since the left ventricle has the greatest pressure most aneurysms occur in the LV
• Develop an akinetic or dyskinetic section of the heart
• See arrhythmias, clots and even obstructive patterns
• ECG changes in an anterior LV aneurysm (can mimic a STEMI)
  • ST elevations V1-V4
  • Non dynamic ST changes
  • Large Q waves in region of old infarct

PERICARDITIS

• Pericardial sac inflammation (without myocardial inflammation)
• Often of viral etiology but can be caused by:
  • Lupus
  • Malignancies
  • Fungal infection
  • HIV
  • Uremia
  • Radiation or chemotherapy
  • Isoniazid or cyclosporin induced
• Chest pain that improves when sitting up and leaning forward
• ECG changes can **progress through four stages:**
  • **Stage 1** – widespread STE and PR depression with reciprocal changes in aVR (occurs during the first two weeks)

- **Stage 2** – normalization of ST changes; generalized T wave flattening (1 to 3 weeks)
- **Stage 3** – flattened T waves become inverted (3 to several weeks)
- **Stage 4** – ECG returns to normal (several weeks onwards)
- Treatment with NSAIDS or Colchicine and generally close outpatient followup

MYOCARDITIS

- Associated viruses (Coxsackie, HIV, Hep C, Chagas)
- Positive troponin (help differentiates myocarditis from pericarditis)
- Variable ECG changes but **often diffuse ST-Twave changes** in a non anatomic distribution
    - Sinus tachycardia.
    - QRS / QT prolongation.
    - Diffuse T wave inversion.
    - Ventricular arrhythmias.
    - AV conduction defects.
- Pericarditis like appearance can occur if there is a *myopericarditis*

ENDOCARDITIS

- Often presents with acute sepsis
- If valvular rupture there is often congestive heart failure
- Unless the patient is a IV drug abuse or has an indwelling venous line it is often involving the **left side of the heart**

Organisms

- Staphylococcus aureus (MSSA or MRSA)
- Coagulase negative Staphylococci: *S. epidermidis, S. lugdenensis*
- Streptococcus viridans
- Streptococcus bovis
- Enterococcus
- HACEK organisms
    - Haemophillus aphrophilus, parainfluenzae and paraphrophilus
    - Actinobacillus actinomycetemcomitans

- Cardiobacterium hominis
  - Eikenella corrodens
  - Kingella kingae
- Fungi

Culture negative endocarditis

- Brucella
- Bartonella
- Coxiella burnetti (Q fever)
- Chlamydia
- Legionella
- Mycoplasma
- Whipples disease (*Trophyerma whipplei*)

Risk Factors

- Congenital heart disease
- Rheumatic heart disease
- Mitral valve prolapse
- Valve regurgitation
- Degenerative valve disease
- Prosthetic valve (1-5%) – early (<60 days) or late (>60 days)
- IV drug use – tricuspid, aortic and mitral valve
- Dialysis
- high risk surgery (e.g. dental, respiratory and infective)
- Indwelling lines such as PICC Lines
- HIV

Exam Findings and Physical Exam

- Hematuria
- Stroke, ICH, and multifocal pneumonia can occur from septic emboli
- Splinter hemorrhages or conjunctival hemorrhages
- Oslers nodes – tender nodules on pulps of fingers and toes
- Janeway lesions – non-tender hemorrhage pulps on fingers and toes
- Roth spots – retinal hemorrhages with a pale centre

- New murmur
- Echocardiography (TTE = 60% sensitive/TEE = 90-99% sensitive, specificity of 90%)

Modified Duke Criteria for diagnosis

- **Two major criteria, or**
- **One major and three minor criteria, or**
- **Five minor criteria**

Major criteria

- Positive blood culture for Infective Endocarditis
  Typical microorganism consistent with IE from 2 separate blood cultures, as noted below:
- Evidence of endocardial involvement
- New valvular regurgitation (worsening or changing of preexisting murmur not sufficient)

Minor criteria

- Predisposing heart condition or intravenous drug use
- Fever: T> 38.0° C (100.4° F)
- Vascular phenomena: major arterial emboli, septic pulmonary infarcts, mycotic aneurysm, intracranial hemorrhage, conjunctival hemorrhages, and Janeway lesions
- Immunologic phenomena: glomerulonephritis, Osler's nodes, Roth spots, and rheumatoid factor
- Positive blood culture consistent with IE
    - Echocardiographic findings consistent with IE
- **IV antibiotics differ based on native or prosthetic valves**

ENDOCARDITIS ANTIBIOTICS

Native Valves

- Ampicillin/Sulbactam 12g/day IV in 4 doses + Gentamicin 3mg/kg/day IV in 2 or 3 doses

Suspected MRSA

- Vancomycin 30mg/kg/day IV in 2 doses and

- Gentamicin 3mg/kg/day IV in 2 or 3 doses and
- Ciprofloxacin 1000mg/day PO in 2 doses or 800 mg/day IV in 2 doses

Prosthetic Valves

- Vancomycin 30mg/kg/day IV in 2 doses and
- Gentamicin 3mg/kg/day IV in 2 or 3 doses and
- Rifampin 1200 mg/day PO in 2 doses

DENTAL PROCEDURE PROPHYLAXIS FOR ENDOCARDITIS

- All antibiotics options are given as a single dose 1 hour prior to the dental procedure.
- In Europe, prophylaxis is no longer recommended and in the U.S. only reserved for those with artificial valves or prior endocarditis
    - Amoxicillin 2g or 50mg/kg PO or
    - Ampicillin 2g (50mg/kg) IV/IM or
    - Clindamycin 600mg (20mg/kg) PO or
    - Azithromycin or Clarithromycin 500mg (15mg/kg) PO

PERICARDIAL TAMPONADE

- **Beck's Triad A collection of three medical signs associated with acute cardiac tamponade**
    - Hypotension with a narrowed pulse pressure
    - Jugular venous distention
    - Muffled heart sounds
- ECG findings
    - Low voltage
    - Electrical alternans (QRS is alternating small and large from beat to beat)
- U/S shows RV collapsing under pressure from effusion
- If traumatic pericardial tamponade, then thoracotomy is indicated
- If non traumatic then a pericardiocentesis is indicated

PERIPHERAL VASCULAR DISEASE

- ABI < 0.90 is consistent with PVD
- Exam can show loss of hair
    - Shiny skin
    - Reduced pulses
    - Ulcers
- At any point extreme PVD can progress to wet or dry gangrene, or acute ulcerative lesions
- **Gas Gangrene**
    - Requires operative debridement and IV antibiotics targeted at Staph, Strep, and anaerobes

ACUTE LIMB ISCHEMIA

The 6 "P's"

- Pain
- Pallor
- Paresthesias
- Perishingly cold
- Pulselessness
- Paralysis

Causes

- 15% likelihood of embolic events from either heart or a AAA
- Acute aortic dissection
- Extensive DVT

Diagnosis and Treatment

- Ultrasound or angiography is needed to confirm location and degree of occluded venous and arterial vasculature
- Empiric anticoagulation is needed during workup followed by embolectomy or thrombolysis

HEART FAILURE

Diastolic Failure

- Long standing HTN causes ventricle hypertrophy and constriction

- This impairs relaxation which impairs diastolic filling
- CHF symptoms but a normal ejection fraction
- Treatment often involves decreasing the heart rate to allow for improved filling

Low output heart failure

- Most common form of failure often caused by:
    - **Ischemic heart disease impairing the ejection fraction**
    - **Cardiomyopathy**
- Present with pulmonary edema if left sided
- Present with JVD and peripheral edema and hepatic congestion if right sided
- BNP - some usefulness to rule out CHF if BNP is normal but BNP elevation can occur for many reasons besides CHF.
- **Treatment**
    - Preload reduction with nitrates
    - Loop diuretics after initial stabilization due to delayed effects
    - Positive pressure ventilation to recruit alveoli in setting of pulmonary edema
    - Decrease after-load with ACEIs
    - Increase contractility with inotropes such as dobutamine

High Output Failure

- Excessive demands on cardiac output that the heart cannot achieve through its ejection fraction and is often caused by:
- Hyperthyroidism
- AV shunts
- Anemia
- Vasodilation from severe burns, beri beri (B1 deficiency) or anaphylaxis/ acute drug reaction

LEFT VENTRICULAR ASSIST DEVICES

- Patients receive LVADS as a bridge to a heart transplant or as a final therapeutic option for severe heart failure ("destination therapy)

LVAD Flow direction

- LVAD — LV to aorta
- RVAD — RA or RV to pulmonary artery
- BiVAD — combination of both of the above
- Due to the non continuous flow (non pulsatile) of the LVAD, normal blood pressure cuffs will not detect a pulse
  - Measure MAP with a doppler (goal 70-90 mmHg)
- **Patients are both preload and after-load sensitive**

Complications

- **Bleeding - most common reason for ED visit**
  - GI Bleed, epistaxis, ICH, intrathoracic bleeding
  - Acquired Von Willebrand Disease (vWD)
  - Supra-therapeutic anticoagulation
  - Lack of pulsatile flow → AV malformations in GI tract
- **Infection**
  - Driveline and pocket are most common sites
  - Usually gram positive bacteria, but also need to cover for fungal infection
- **Pump Thrombosis**
  - Low output state with falsely elevated pump flow estimates on controller
  - Diagnose with echo or cardiac CTA
  - Treatment with heparin and anti-platelet therapy
  - Consider tPA in life-threatening situations in coordination with VAD team
- **Arrhythmia - very common**
  - Get labs to evaluate electrolytes and troponin
  - Treat atrial fibrillation as in any other patient
  - Treat ventricular arrhythmias with volume replacement and pharmacological or electrical cardioversion
  - Place pads anterior/posterior performing cardioversion or defibrillation
- **Low power warnings** - require new battery or immediate wall power
- Immediately consult VAD team/coordinator

WOLFF-PARKINSON-WHITE SYNDROME

- Accessory pathway from atrium to ventricle with rapid conduction
    - Treatment of regular rate WPW is with adenosine
- WPW with Atrial fibrillation
    - Requires immediate cardioversion as adenosine can block normal condition and cause degeneration to an unstable rhythm.

VENTRICULAR TACHYCARDIA

- Wide complex, regular tachycardia is ventricular tachycardia (VT) until proven otherwise
- SVT with aberrant conduction (a bundle branch block) can mimic VT

TORSADES D POINTES

- Ventricular tachycardia from QT prolongation
- Treat with magnesium acute defibrillation and overdrive pacing

PACEMAKERS AND AICDS

- Historically AICDs were implanted in patients with severe congestive heart failure.
- The majority of devices today are combined devices.
- Magnet held overtop of a pacer sets it into demand mode where it stops sensing and paces at a fixed rate
- **Magnet held overtop of an AICD disables defibrillation and cardioversion**
- Do not defibrillate overtop of an AICD. (place defibrillation pads in anterior lateral positioning)
- A chest X-ray can evaluate for lead fractures post trauma

PULSELESS ELECTRICAL ACTIVITY

"Pump, Pipes, Tank" method

- **Pump Failure**
    - STEMI
    - Tension pneumothorax

- Tamponade
- Hyperkalemia induced dysfunction
- Hypoxia causing cardiac ischemia
- Severe hypovolemia (fluids)
- **Pipe Failure**
  - Circulatory obstruction (PE)
  - Circulatory failure (AAA, dissection, anaphylaxis)
- **Tank Insufficiency**
  - Severe hypovolemia

Traditional H's and T's

- **6 "H's"**
  - Hypovolemia
  - Hypoxia
  - Hydrogen ion (acidosis)
  - Hyper/hypokalemia
  - Hypoglycemia
  - Hypothermia
- **5 "T's"**
  - Toxins
  - Tamponade (cardiac)
  - Tension pneumothorax
  - Thrombosis (coronary and pulmonary)
  - Trauma

WIDE COMPLEX TACHYCARDIA

Regular

- Monomorphic ventricular tachycardia
- PSVT with aberrant conduction:
  - PSVT with bundle branch block^
  - PSVT with accessory pathway
  - Atrial flutter with bundle branch block
- Sinus tachycardia with bundle branch block

- Accelerated idioventricular rhythm (consider if less than or ~120 bpm)
- Metabolic
    - Hyperkalemia
    - Digoxin toxicity
- Severe metabolic acidosis

Irregular

- Atrial fibrillation/atrial flutter with variable AV conduction AND bundle branch block
- Atrial fibrillation/atrial flutter with variable AV conduction AND accessory pathway (e.g. WPW)
- Atrial fibrillation + hyperkalemia
- Polymorphic ventricular tachycardia
    - Torsades de pointes
    - Non-sustained ventricular tachycardia

NARROW COMPLEX TACHYCARDIA

Regular

- AV Node Independent
    - Sinus tachycardia
    - Atrial tachycardia (uni-focal or multi-focal)
    - Atrial fibrillation
    - Atrial flutter
- AV Node Dependent
    - Paroxysmal supraventricular tachycardia (PSVT)
    - AV node re-entry tachycardia (AVNRT)
    - AV re-entry tachycardia (AVRT)
    - Lown-Ganong-Levine syndrome
    - Wolff–Parkinson–White syndrome
    - Junctional tachycardia

Irregular

- Multifocal atrial tachycardia (MAT)
- Sinus tachycardia with frequent PACs

- Atrial fibrillation
- Atrial flutter with variable conduction

SUPRAVENTRICULAR TACHYCARDIA (SVT)

- SVT is a collective term that refers to any arrythmia originating above the ventricle. This includes
  - Sinus tachycardia
  - Atrioventricular node re-entrant tachycardia (AVNRT)
    - Treat with calcium channel blockers or adenosine
  - Atrioventricular reciprocating tachycardia (AVRT)
    - Treat with calcium channel blockers or adenosine
  - Atrial fibrillation
  - Atrial flutter
  - Multifocal atrial tachycardia

HYPERTENSIVE EMERGENCY

- **Hypertensive Emergency = Hypertension and one of the following**

Intracranial hemorrhage

- **SAH -** Decrease blood pressure and prevent vasospasm with nimodipine
- **Intraparencymal hemorrhage -** Lower blood pressure with nicardipine

Preeclampsia/Eclampsia

- Treat with magnesium and lower blood pressure with labetolol or hydralazine

Cardiac/Vascular disruption

- **ACS/pulmonary edema -** decrease preload with nitrates
- **Acute aortic dissection** - decrease shear forces with beta blockade and then lower blood pressure with nicardipine or nitropruside.

Alpha Crisis

- **Pheochromocytoma's** - provide alpha blockade (phentolamine)
- **MAOI overdose** - supportive care

- **Sympathomimetics such as cocaine and amphetamines** - provide supportive care and avoid beta-blockade due to feared theoretically unposed alpha stimulation that can occur

Dermatology

SMALL LESIONS (<0.5CM)

- Macule – flat, circumscribed, colored, non palpable
- Papule – raised, solid and palpable
- Vesicle – raised, palpable, clear fluid-filled
- Pustule – raised, palpable, pus filled (leukocytes or keratin)

LARGE LESIONS (>0.5CM)

- Patch – large macule (flat non-palpable colored area)
- Plaque – superficially raised, circumscribed solid area
- Nodule – distinct large papule
- Bulla - large vesicle (blisters if epidermal layer completely sloughed off)
- Wheal – firm and edematous plaque (edema of the dermis)

ABSCESS AND CELLULITIS

- **Cellulitis** - erythematous painful epidermis - treat with oral antibiotics
  - Outpatient Treatment
    - Cephalexin
    - Macrolide
    - Amoxicillin/clavulanic acid
- **Abscess** - Fluctuant region with or without associated cellulitis (most often Staph species)
  - I&D is definitive treatment
  - Antibiotics with MRSA coverage may prevent complications:
    - TMP-SMX
    - Clindamycin
    - Doxycycline
- Consider admission and IV antibiotics if
  - **Outpatient therapy fails**
  - **Immunocompromised**

- **Sympathomimetics such as cocaine and amphetamines** - provide supportive care and avoid beta-blockade due to feared theoretically unposed alpha stimulation that can occur

Dermatology

SMALL LESIONS (<0.5CM)

- Macule – flat, circumscribed, colored, non palpable
- Papule – raised, solid and palpable
- Vesicle – raised, palpable, clear fluid-filled
- Pustule – raised, palpable, pus filled (leukocytes or keratin)

LARGE LESIONS (>0.5CM)

- Patch – large macule (flat non-palpable colored area)
- Plaque – superficially raised, circumscribed solid area
- Nodule – distinct large papule
- Bulla - large vesicle (blisters if epidermal layer completely sloughed off)
- Wheal – firm and edematous plaque (edema of the dermis)

ABSCESS AND CELLULITIS

- **Cellulitis** - erythematous painful epidermis - treat with oral antibiotics
    - Outpatient Treatment
        - Cephalexin
        - Macrolide
        - Amoxicillin/clavulanic acid
- **Abscess** - Fluctuant region with or without associated cellulitis (most often Staph species)
    - I&D is definitive treatment
    - Antibiotics with MRSA coverage may prevent complications:
        - TMP-SMX
        - Clindamycin
        - Doxycycline
- Consider admission and IV antibiotics if
    - **Outpatient therapy fails**
    - **Immunocompromised**

ERYSIPELAS

- Similar to cellulitis but more superficial with clear demarcations (often raised edges) with a fast onset and greater systemic effects (fever, mild sepsis) caused by:
    - Beta hemolytic strep (most common)
    - H. influenza (in unimmunized children)

Antibiotic Options

- Penicillin G 300K U/d IM for <30 kg, 600K to 1 million U/d IM for >30 kg (first line therapy) or
- Clindamycin 450mg (5mg/kg) PO q8hrs x 10 days (if PCN allergic) or
- Cephalexin 500mg (6.25mg/kg) PO q6hrs x 10 days or
- Ceftriaxone 1g (50mg/kg) IV once daily x 10 days or
- Levofloxacin 500mg PO/IV daily x 10 days or
- Augmentin 500mg PO BID x 10 days (generally reserved for failure of first line therapy)
- Bullous Erysipelas or MRSA suspected: trimethoprim-sulfamethoxazole, clindamycin, doxycycline, or minocycline

ERYTHEMATOUS RASH DIFFERENTIAL

Positive Nikolsky's sign and

- **Febrile**
    - Staphylococcal scalded skin syndrome (children)
    - Toxic epidermal necrolysis (adults)
- **Afebrile**
    - Toxic epidermal necrolysis

Negative Nikolsky's sign

- **Febrile**
    - Toxic shock syndrome
    - Kawasaki disease
    - Scarlet fever
- **Afebrile**
    - Anaphylaxis

- Scombroid
- Alcohol intoxication

IMPETIGO

- Group A strep or staph species caused superficial skin infection
- Often in children age 205 years old
- Treat with topical antibiotics: Mupirocin
- Oral antibiotics rarely needed (penicillins and cephalosporins)

STAPH SCALDED SKIN SYNDROME (SSS)

- Staph exotoxin mediated systemic process
- Rash progresses from erythroderma to extensive areas of exfoliation
- Systemic symptoms (malaise, fever, irritability, skin tenderness) are common
- Nikolsky's sign (separation of epidermis when pressure is applied) is present
- No mucous membrane involvement (differentiate from SJS/TENS)
- Treat with **clindamycin** to inhibit the causative exotoxin and kill the Staph.

TOXIC SHOCK SYNDROME

- Most commonly from S. aureus strain produces toxic shock syndrome toxin-1 (super-antigen) is the most common cause
- Group A strep. is a less common cause

Clinical Criteria Staphylococcal toxic shock

- **Fever**: temperature >38.9°C
- **Rash**: diffuse macular erythroderma
- **Hypotension**: systolic blood pressure <90 mm Hg (adults) or <5th percentile for age (children younger than 16 years), or orthostatic hypotension, dizziness, or syncope
- **Multisystem dysfunction:**
    - Gastrointestinal: vomiting or diarrhea at onset of illness
    - Muscular: severe myalgias, or serum creatine phosphokinase level (CPK) greater than twice the upper limit of normal

- Mucous membranes: vaginal, oropharyngeal, or conjunctival hyperemia
- Renal: blood urea nitrogen or creatinine level greater than twice the upper limit of normal, or pyuria (5 leukocytes per high-power field), in the absence of urinary tract infection
- Hepatic: total serum bilirubin or transaminase level greater than twice the upper limit of normal
- Hematologic: platelets <100,000/L
- Central nervous system: disorientation or alteration in consciousness but no focal neurologic signs at a time when fever and hypotension are absent.
- Desquamation: One to 2 weeks after the onset of illness (typically palms and soles)

VESICULOBULLOUS RASHES

Differential diagnosis if Febrile

- **Diffuse distribution**
  - Varicella
  - Smallpox
  - Disseminated gonococcal disease
  - DIC
- **Localized distribution**
  - Necrotizing fasciitis
  - Hand-foot-and-mouth disease

Differential diagnosis if afebrile

- **Diffuse distribution**
  - Bullous pemphigoid (less mucous membrane involvement than P. vulgaris)
  - Drug-Induced bullous disorders
  - Pemphigus vulgaris (higher mortality than bullous pemphigoid)
  - Phytophotodermatitis
  - Erythema multiforme major
- **Localized distribution**

- Contact dermatitis
- Herpes zoster
- Burn
- Dermatitis herpetiformis
- Erythema multiforme minor
- Poison Oak, Ivy, Sumac dermatitis
- Bullosis diabeticorum

STEVENS-JOHNSON SYNDROME (SJS) & TOXIC EPIDERMAL NECROLYSIS (TEN)

- SJS and TEN exist on a spectrum of disease
- SJS involves <10% of body surface area
- TEN involves >30% of body surface area
- Both often have a Nikolsky sign (denude when touched)
- In severe cases, respiratory tract and GI involvement may occur
- Fluid replacement - treat shock with IV fluids according to burn protocols

Causes

- **Medications**
- **HIV**
- **Malignancies (lymphoma)**

Treatment

- **Treat as burn with fluid resuscitation and ICU level supportive care**

FUNGAL INFECTIONS

- Tinea infections are caused by richophyton, Epidermophyton, Microsporum
  - **Tinea Pedis** - involves the feet
  - **Tinea manus** - involving the feet
  - **Tinea capitis** - involving the scalp
  - **Tinea cruris** - involving the groin
- **Intertrigo** - involves skin folds (commonly from candida spp.)

- **Onychomycosis** - involving the nails
- For all the above infections topical "azoles" such as clotrimazole often fully treat the condition within weeks if paired with good skin hygiene (dry and clean)
- **Kerions**:
  - Scalp plaques caused by ringworm
  - Broken hair follicles and associated baldness at the region of greatest fungal infection
  - Requires 8-week course of oral griseofulvin contrary to epidermis associated ringworm which can receive topical therapy
- **Thrush**:
  - **Candidal** infection of the oropharynx with associated surrounding edema
  - plaques scrape off (contrast to leukoplakia associated with EBV and HIV)
  - **Oral anti-fungals** (nystatin) provides treatment within a week provided the patient is no immunocompromised

HERPES ZOSTER

Varicella zoster reactivation

- Highly contagious until lesions crust
- Symptoms start with prodrome of pain followed by dermatomal distribution vesicular rash
- Treatment: oral acyclovir (except in disseminated cases)
- Hutchinson's sign (nasal lesions) - a sign of Herpes ophthalmicus which should prompt corneal staining in the ED to evaluation fo ulcerations or perforations
- Ramsay-Hunt syndrome - vesicular lesions on ear
  - Greater association with facial nerve paralysis and vertigo

Disseminated zoster

- Unlike normal zoster, disseminated zoster will cross midline and involve > 3 dermatomes
- Generally only occurs in the immunocompromised patients
- Complications include hepatitis, pneumonitis, encephalitis,

- IV acyclovir

MOLLUSCUM CONTAGIOSUM

- Papules with an umbilicated center
- Painless, self resolving, most often in children due to viral exposure
- Widespread lesions in an adult should prompt an HIV test

HUMAN PAPILLOMAVIRUS

- **Condyloma acuminata (warts):**
    - Flesh colored cauliflower like growths in genital/perianal areas
    - Usually painless but can bleed
- Vaccines target the cancer causing strains of HPV since there are over 40 subtypes (most not oncogenic)
- Topical anesthetics can provide pain relief for short courses

SCABIES

- Infestation with the *Sarcoptes scabiei* mite (an ectoparasite)
- 4-6 week incubation period after initial exposure
- Norwegian scabies - Severe disease with diffuse scabies
- Treatment:
- **Permethrin** 5% cream for all household members
    - Apply from neck down and Leave on for 8-12hr before washing off
- **Ivermectin** 200 mcg/kg may be necessary for severe infection
    - Contraindicated in lactating women and children < 15kg

OTHER ECTOPARASITES

- Bed bugs, Lice, Myiasis, Scabies, Ticks

ERYTHEMA MULTIFORME

- Acute, self-limited skin condition identified by Erythematous Target lesions with "three zones of color" (may be HSV related)

Erythema multiforme minor

- Typical targets or raised, edematous papules distributed peripherally
- No mucous membrane involvement

Erythema multiforme major

- Same as EM minor + involvement of 1+ mucous membranes
- Epidermal detachment involves < 10% of total body surface area
- Some cases can be severe or even fatal
- Treatment is symptomatic therapy (antihistamines)

DECUBITUS ULCERS

- All ulcers place the patient at risk for osteomyelitis and sepsis although most common in stage 3-4 wounds
    - Stage 1 - Epidermal redness only
    - Stage 2 - Erosion into epidermis only (dermis is intact)
    - Stage 3 - Deep necrosis/ulceration to all skin layers above fascia
    - Stage 4 - Full thickness ulceration revealing muscle and bone

URTICARIA

- Type 1 hypersensitivity reaction
- Less severe than anaphylaxis (only skin manifestations)
- Treat with Histamine antagonists to improve symptoms

ECZEMA HERPETICUM

- HSV super-infected eczema
- Development of vesicular eruptions containing HSV 1 or 2 in areas of epidermis previously affected by atopic dermatitis
- Multiple organ systems can be involved, resulting in lymphadenopathy, keratoconjunctivitis and resulting blindness, meningitis, encephalitis.

PITYRIASIS ROSEA

- Mild inflammatory exanthem that starts with a "herald patch" (isolated 2-5cm oval lesion)
- May be caused by HHV 6 and 7
- 70% preceded by URI

- Most common 10-35yr old
- Not contagious
- Spontaneous resolution occurs within 4-12wk

PSORIASIS

- Psoriasis is a chronic and relapsing disease treated with topical corticosteroids (hydrocortisone cream 1-2%)
- **Plaque:** also known as psoriasis vulgaris, makes up about 90% of cases. It typically presents as red patches with white scales on top. Areas of the body most commonly affected are the back of the forearms, shins, navel area, and scalp.
- **Guttate:** drop-shaped lesions.
- **Inverse:** red patches in skin folds
- **Pustular:** presents as small non-infectious pus-filled blisters
- **Erythrodermic:** occurs when the rash becomes very widespread, and can develop from any of the other types. Fingernails and toenails are affected in most people with psoriasis at some point in time. This may include pits in the nails or changes in nail color.

SEBACEOUS CYST

- Obstruction of a hair follicle causing sebum accumulation which can develop an abscess
- Treat with I&D with capsule removal if possible to prevent recurrence.

CELLULITIS/SUPERFICIAL ABSCESS WITH CELLULITIS

- Tailor antibiotics by regional antibiogram

Outpatient

- Coverage primarily for Strep
- MRSA coverage only necessary if cellulitis associated with: purulence, penetrating trauma, known MRSA colonization, IV drug use, or SIRS
- 5 day treatment duration, unless symptoms do not improve within that timeframe

- Cephalexin 500mg PO q6hrs or
- Add TMP/SMX DS 1 tab PO BID if MRSA is suspected
- Most cases of non-purulent cellulitis are caused by Strep. In these cases, the addition of TMP/SMX has been demonstrated to offer no clinical benefit over cephalexin alone.
- Clindamycin 450mg PO TID covers both Strep and Staph
- Tetracyclines (like Doxycycline) should be avoided in non-purulent cellulitis due to high rates of Strep resistance

Inpatient

- Vancomycin 20mg/kg IV q12hrs or
- Clindamycin 600mg IV q8hrs or
- Linezolid 600mg IV q12hrs or
- Daptomycin 4mg/kg IV once daily

Saltwater related cellulitis

- coverage extended for Vibrio vulnificus
- Doxycycline 100mg PO/IV q12hrs daily and Cefepime 1g IV q12hrs x 10 days
- Ciprofloxacin 400mg IV q12hrs x 10 days
- Ciprofloxacin 750mg PO q12hrs x 10 days

Freshwater related cellulitis

- coverage extended for Aeromonas
- Ciprofloxacin 400mg IV q12hrs x 10 days
- Ciprofloxacin 500mg PO q12hrs x 10 days
- TMP/SMX 2 DS tablets (5mg/kg) PO q12hrs x 10 days
- Ceftriaxone 1g (50mg/kg) IV q24hrs

IMPETIGO

- Coverage for MSSA, MRSA, Group A Strep

Topical therapy

- Mupirocin (Bactroban) 2% ointment q8hrs x 5 days
- For non-bullous impetigo, topic antibiotics are as effective as oral antibiotics

Oral Therapy

- Cephalexin 500mg (6.25mg/kg) PO q6hrs for 10 days or
- Amoxicillin/Clavulanate 875mg (12.5mg/kg) PO q12hrs daily x 10 days or
- Clindamycin 450mg PO q8hrs daily (or 10mg/kg PO q6hrs) for 10 days or
- Dicloxacillin 500mg (3mg/kg) PO q6hrs daily x 10 days

EMS

EMERGENCY MEDICAL TREATMENT AND ACTIVE LABOR ACT (EMTALA)

- Regardless of patient's ability to pay or insurance status, an emergency department must perform a medical screening exam to determine if an emergent condition exists or patient is in active labor.
- Hospital is obligated to stabilize the patient. If the hospital is unable to provide the necessary care after stabilization, then the sending physician must find a facility that can provide necessary care.

RYAN WHITE COMPREHENSIVE AIDS RESOURCES EMERGENCY (CARE) ACT OF 1990

- Also known as the Ryan White Act
- Required that each agency have an infection control officer. Reporting is mandatory when:
    - Emergency response employee believes an exposure has occurred.
    - Health Care facility identifies an infectious and transmissible agent.

EMS SYSTEM TYPES

- **Fire-Based** - Traditional integration with fire departments.
- **Hospital-Based** -Less common, with hospital training, staffing and maintaining EMS.
- **Private** - Corporate entity manages the EMS agency, with various levels of government oversight or involvement. Often perform inter-facility transports of BLS responses
- **Third Service** - Fire and Police are the first two services. EMS exists separately and controls its own budget, staffing, and priorities.
- **Public Utility** - Similar to the gas and electric company. Local government establishes an EMS Authority that contracts with a private company

- **Volunteer Systems** - More common in rural systems. Often organized as not for profit charitable corporations 501(c)(3).

MEDICAL CONTROL

- **Offline (Indirect)** - standing orders and protocolized care
- **Online (Direct)** - augmentation of protocolized care with direct physician communication (can also be on-scene care if a physician is present)

PROVIDER SKILL LEVELS

Emergency Medicine Responder (EMR)

- BLS skills

Emergency Medicine Technician (EMT)

- BLS skills plus oral med administration (aspirin, glucose)

Advanced Emergency Medical Technician (AEMT)

- BLS skills, some IV and IM medications

Paramedic

- All of the above skills + IV medications and more advance medical knowledge such as ECG interpretation and transcutaneous pacing.
- Endotracheal Intubation

MASS CASUALTY TRIAGE CATEGORIES

- Red - critical
- Yellow - delayed
- Green - minor ("walking wounded")
- Black - expectant or dead (level 4)
- Patients are triaged first by those who can walk from the area unassisted (minor injuries), then the Red (critical patients) who need immediate care, and finally the patients with intermediate injuries who can wait for delayed care.

PHASES OF DISASTER CARE

- Preparedness
- Response
- Recover
- Mitigation

TRAUMA CENTER LEVEL DESIGNATIONS

- Level 1 - all subspecialties available 24/7 + research funding
- Level II - some subspecialties but 24/7 trauma surgery
- Level III - ED capabilities with surgery on-call
- Level IV - ED capabilities but minimal on call assistance and no guaranteed surgical subspecialties

Endocrinology

GENERAL ACID BASE APPROACH

- Primary acidosis if pH <7.38
- HCO3 <24 = metabolic acidosis
- Always determine if there is another acid/base process occurring
- Primary respiratory acidosis if pCO2 > pCO2expected
- Primary respiratory alkalosis if pCO2 < pCO2expected
    - use Winter's formula: PCO2 (expected) = (1.5 x [HCO3–] + 8) ± 2
    - In acute setting PCO2 should fall by 1 mmHg for every 1 mEq fall in HCO3
- Concurrent metabolic alkalosis if delta-delta > 28
    - Delta-Delta = (AG - 12) + HCO3

ANION GAP

- Anion gap = Na - (Cl + HCO3)

WINTERS FORMULA

- Used to assess respiratory compensation in response to a metabolic acidosis
- Expected PCO2 = 1.5 x HCO3 + 8 if there is adequate compensation

OSMOL GAP

- **Osm gap = measured osm - calculated osm (normal 10-15)**
- 2(Na)+glucose/18) +(BUN/2.8) + (Blood alcohol level/5)

ANION GAP METABOLIC ACIDOSIS

- MUDPILESCAT (**M**ethanol, **U**remia, **D**KA, **P**henformin (**p**aracetamol), **I**NH or **I**ron, **L**actic acidosis, **E**thylene glycol, **S**alicylates, **C**arbon monoxide or **C**yanide poisoning, **A**lcohol ketoacidosis, **T**oluene)

Lactic acidosis

- Sepsis, shock, liver disease, CO, CN, metformin, methemoglobin

- Short bowel syndrome

Renal failure

- Uremia

Ketoacidosis

- DKA
- Alcoholic Ketoacidosis
- Starvation ketoacidosis

Ingestions

- Acetaminophen toxicity
- Aspirin toxicity
- Increased osm gap
    - Methanol
    - Ethylene glycol
- Normal osm gap
    - Salicylate toxicity
    - Iron
    - INH

NON-ANION GAP METABOLIC ACIDOSIS

Hyperkalemia

- Resolving DKA
- Early uremic acidosis
- Early obstructive uropathy
- RTA Type IV
- Hypoaldosteronism
- K-sparing diuretics

Hypokalemia

- RTA Type I
- RTA Type II
- Acetazolamide

- Acute diarrhea

Hyperchloremic IVF infusions

Hyperalimentation

RESPIRATORY ACIDOSIS

- **Respiratory acidosis = pCO2 > 42**

Differential diagnosis (primarily hypoventilation)

- **COPD/Asthma**
    - Treat with steroids, bronchodilators, alveolar recruitment (CPAP/Bipap)
- **Opioid overdose**
    - Treat with reversal (naloxone) and respiratory support
- **Severe Trauma**
    - Resuscitation and correction of surgical pathology
- **Treatment is focused at improving ventilation specific to the underlying disease**

METABOLIC ALKALOSIS

- Metabolic alkalosis generally occurs as a primary increase in serum bicarbonate concentration (contraction alkalosis), which can occur due to loss of H+ from the body or a gain in HCO3-.
    - Primary causes are diuretic overuse and GI volume loss via vomiting or diarrhea
    - Treatment is mainly fluid repletion and correction of other associated electrolyte losses.
- Also associated with hypokalemia and hypocalcemia (causing global weakness)

RESPIRATORY ALKALOSIS

- Most often respiratory alkalosis is a response to an underlying metabolic acidosis in an attempt to compensate.
- Hyperventilation (anxiety, aspirin toxicity) is the most common cause of a primary respiratory alkalosis

ADRENAL INSUFFICIENCY

Primary adrenal insufficiency (decreased cortisol and aldosterone production)

- Autoimmune (70%)
- Adrenal hemorrhage
    - Coagulation disorders
    - Sepsis (Waterhouse-Friderichsen syndrome)
- Medication related (excessive steroid use)
- TB (most common worldwide)
- Sarcoidosis/amyloidosis
- Congenital adrenal hyperplasia

Secondary adrenal insufficiency (decreased ACTH → decreases cortisol production)

- Withdrawal of steroid therapy
- Pituitary disease
- Head trauma
- Postpartum pituitary necrosis
- Infiltrative disorders of pituitary or hypothalamus

Clinical Presentation

- Hypotension (refractory to fluids/vasopressors)
- Hyponatremia/Hyperkalemia (hyperkalemia is not expected in secondary adrenal insufficiency)
- Hypoglycemia
- Dehydration
- Abdominal tenderness
- Confusion/delirium/lethargy
- Hyperpigmentation (Primary insufficiency/Addison's disease)
- Treat with stress-dose steroid (hydrocortisone or fludrocortisone)

RELATIVE POTENCY OF STEROID FORMULATIONS

Steroid Name	Glucocorticoid Activity	Mineralocorticoid Activity
Hydrocortisone	1	1
Prednisolone	4	0.8
Dexamethasone	30	None
Fludrocortisone	10	125

CUSHING'S SYNDROME

- Hypercortisolism caused by excess **steroid ingestion or ACTH secreting tumors**
- **Metabolic: hypokalemia, hypochloremia and hyperglycemia**
- Soft Tissue: proximal muscle atrophy, weakness, progressive obesity (buffalo hump/supraclavicular fat pads)
- Ophthalmologic: cataracts, increased intraocular pressure
- Bone: osteoporosis
- Psychologic: emotional lability, depression, irritability, anxiety, panic attacks, mild paranoia and mania

HYPERCALCEMIA

Causes:

- Malignancy, Hyperparathyroidism, Lithium, Thiazides, Hypothyroidism, Addison's, Sarcoid, Hyperthyroid, Excess vitamin D ingestion
- **"Stones"**
    - Renal calculi
    - Renal failure
- **"Bones"**
    - Bone pain/destruction
- **"Groans"**
    - Abdominal pain, vomiting
    - Dehydration
    - Pancreatitis
- **"Thrones"**
    - Polyuria/polydipsia (Renal insufficiency)

- Constipation
- **"Psychic Overtones"**
  - Lethargy/confusion/Hallucinations
- Treat with fluids and loop diuretics while evaluating underlying potential causes

HYPOCALCEMIA

- Corrected Ca = (0.8 *(Normal Alb - Patient's Alb)) + Serum CaDiabetic Ketoacidosis
  - 15% bound to anions (phosphate, lactate, citrate)
  - 40% bound to albumin
  - 45% free (regulated by PTH, Vit-D)

Signs and Symptoms

- Prolonged QT
- Ckvostek's sign (Facial nerve spasm)
- Trousseau's sign (carpopedal spasm)
- Hyperreflexia
- Seizures

Causes

- Pancreatitis
- Hypomagnesemia
- Rhabdomyolysis (phosphate binds calcium)
- Massive transfusion
- Systemic Hydrofluoric Acid toxicity

Decreased absorption

- Vitamin D deficiency
- Increased excretion
- Alcoholism
- Renal Failure
- Diuretics

Endocrine

- Hypoparathyroidism

Drug adverse events

HYPERGLYCEMIC HYPEROSMOLAR NON-KETOSIS

- Glucose > 1000 mg/dL
- Mild ketonemia (less than DKA)
- Require substantial more fluid resuscitation than patients in DKA in addition to an insulin drip Hypoglycemia

DIABETIC KETOACIDOSIS

- Glucose > 250mg/dl, acidosis (pH < 7.3), and ketonemia
- Multifactorial but major causes include
  - Acute infection
  - Inadequate insulin use
  - Pregnancy
  - Severe trauma
  - Acute myocardial infarct

Treatment

- Volume repletion with 20-30cc/kg isotonic bolus during the first hour
- Check metabolic panel ever 2 hours and blood glucose ever 1 hour
- If potassium <3.5mEq/L, do not administer insulin until potassium supplementation since insulin will shift K intracellularly
- A bolus dose is unnecessary and may contribute to increased hypoglycemic episodes
- Initial infusion 0.1units/kg/hr of insulin
- Add D5 or D10 infusions when blood glucose drops below 250mg/dL
- Continue insulin infusion until anion gap bicarb normalizes
- Alternative subcutaneous regimens utilize short acting insulin (aspart) at 0.3units/kg as initial dosing followed by 0.1units/kg per hour

HYPOMAGNESEMIA

- Impacts potassium absorption and is affected by calcium and phosphorus levels

- Symptoms of lethargy, weakness, and seizures
- Treat symptomatic patients with magnesium sulfate infusions (1-2g/hr)

HYPERMAGNESEMIA

- Treat severe toxicity with 200 mg IV and consider dialysis.
- Treat mild to moderate symptoms with hydration and cessation of exogenous magnesium

Toxicity by magnesium levels

- 2-3 mg/dL - Vomitting
- 3-4 mg/dL - Lethargy
- 4-8 mg/dL - Loss of reflexes
- 8-12 mg/dL - Respiratory depression
- 12-15 mg/dL - Shock, cardiac arrest

HYPOPHOSPHATEMIA

- Presents with weakness and encephalopathy at levels < 1.0mg/dL
- Caused by renal losses or GI malabsorption
- Treat with oral replacement for mild symptoms and IV infusion (KPhos 2.5-5mg/kg IV over 6hr) for severe weakness/paralysis

HYPERPHOSPHATEMIA

- Severe symptoms occur with hyperphosphatemia > 14 mg/dl with moderate symptoms > 4.5 mg/dL

Causes

- Vitamin D intoxication
- Tumor lysis syndrome
- Laxative (Phospho-soda) abuse
- Rhabdomyolysis
- Hypoparathyroidism
- Pseudohypoparathyroidism
- Multiple myeloma

Treatment

- Treat the underlying process
- Restrict calcium phosphate intake
- IV Normal Saline
- Acetazolamide (500mg IV q6hr) - if normal renal function
- Phosphate Binder (Aluminum hydroxide 50-150mg/kg PO q4-6h)

HYPOKALEMIA

- Symptoms can occur with K < 2.5 mEq/L and often due to renal or GI losses
- Every 10mEq KCl increases serum K by approximately 0.1mEq/L
- Rate of IV infusion should not exceed 10mEq/hr to minimize cardiac toxicity
- Preference should always be given to oral repletion
- Also evaluate and treat concomitant hypomagnesemia
- ECG changes: U waves, flat T waves, ST depressions

HYPERKALEMIA

- K > 5.5 mEq/L

Causes

- Hemolyzed sample (pseudohyperkalemia)
- Renal failure
- Exogenous K

ECG changes (often when K > 6.5 mEq/L) often not sequential in progression

- Peaked T-waves
- Bradycardia
- P wave flattening
- QRS prolongation
- Sine Wave
- V. fib
- 2nd and 3rd degree heart blocks

Stabilize the cardiac membrane

- Calcium gluconate: 3 gm over 10 mins
  - Only 1/3 the calcium compared to calcium chloride
- Calcium chloride 1 gram IV over 2-5 minutes
  - Extravasation is caustic so ensure stable IV or central line
  - Effect in 15-30 minutes and duration up to 50 minutes

Shift K+ intracellularly

- **Intravenous insulin (5-10 units regular insulin) + dextrose (50ml of 50% dextrose)**
  - Duration of effect: 4 - 6 hours
  - Decrease the dose to 5units of insulin for renal failure patients due to delayed clearance I
- **Nebulized albuterol 10 - 20mg**
  - Peak effect: 30 minutes
  - Duration of effect: 2 hours
- **Intravenous sodium bicarbonate 50ml of 8.4% solution (1 ampoule) given over 5 minutes**
  - Duration of effect: 1 - 2 hours
  - Generally not required, unless pH <7.1

Excrete K+ from body

- **Intravenous furosemide (Lasix) 40 - 80mg**
  - Ensure adequate urine output first
- **Sodium polystyrene sulfonate (Kayexalate): 30 gm oral or per rectum**
  - Very Controversial, High Risk of Bowel Perforation with sorbitol preparations
- **Sodium zirconium cyclosilicate**
  - Potassium binder, similar to Kayexalate with possibly greater safety profile
- **Definitive treatment by hemodialysis**

HYPONATREMIA

- Patients often not symptomatic until <120meq/L and should be limited to a correction of 10 mEq/L per 24hr (to avoid osmotic demyelination syndrome)

Hypovolemic

- Thiazide diuretic use
- Na-wasting nephroathy (RTA, CRF)
- Osmotic diuresis (glucose, urea)
- Aldosterone deficiency
- GI loss
- 3rd space loss
- Burns
- Pancreatitis

Hypervolemic

- Urinary Na >20 implies renal losses
- Urinary Na <20 implies volume dilution via nephrotic syndrome, cirrhosis, congestive heart-failure

Euvolemic

- SIADH - urine sodium is greater than 20-40 mEq/L
- Psychogenic polydipsia
- Hypothyroidism or Adrenal insufficiency
- Beer podomania (excessive free water intake)

Pseudohyponatremia

- Hyperglycemia
    - Na+ decreases by 2.4mEq/L for each 100mg/dL increase in glucose over 100mg/dL
- Hyperlipidemia and Hyperproteinemia interfere with Na+ estimation by the lab

Hyponatremic induced seizures

- 3% hypertonic saline 150 mL bolus over 20 min (max 3 doses)
- Immediate check sodium after administration of 3% sodium

HYPERNATREMIA

- Na > 145 mEq/L
- Almost entirely from excessive free water loss

- Avoid correction of 10-15 mEq/L/day
- Free water deficit = (0.6 x wt in kg) x [(serum Na/140) – 1]
- Each liter free water deficit increases Na by 3-5 meq/L

THYROID STORM

- The between severe thyrotoxicosis and thyroid storm is a clinical diagnosis and the Burch & Wartofsky diagnostic criteria can predict the likelihood of thyroid storm.
- Classic triad: **hyperthermia, tachycardia, and altered mental status.**

Treat adrenergic tone

- Propranolol PO 60-80 mg q4hr (if can tolerate PO)
- Propranolol IV 1-2mg over 10 min; if tolerates then 1-2mg boluses q15 minutes until HR <100
- Propranolol also partially blocks conversion of T3 to T4

Block Hormone Synthesis

- **PTU 500-1000mg PO or NG followed by 250mg q4hr**
    - Note black box warning of hepatotoxicity so check LFTs prior
- **Methimazole 20-25mg q4hr (80 - 100 mg daily in divided doses)**
    - Longer acting than PTU
    - Should be avoided in pregnancy
- **Potassium iodide (SSKI)**
    - Give 1hr after PTU or methimazole to prevent increased hormone production (Jod-Basedow effect)
    - Block hormone release: (Wolff-Chaikoff effect) only after hormone synthesis is inhibited. Iodine concentration leads to transient decrease of T3/T4
- **Lithium carbonate**
    - Consider if iodine allergic
    - Lithium carbonate 300mg PO q8hr
    - Treatment of choice for iodine-induced hyperthyroidism as the result of contrast load or amiodarone
- Lugol's Solution 8 drops PO q 6 (alternative iodine source)
- Sodium Iodide 0.5mg IV Q 12 hours (alternative iodine source)

Adrenal Insufficiency (often associated with thyroid storm)

- Hydrocortisone 300mg IV bolus, followed by 100mg TID for several days

Plasmapheresis

- Reserved for extreme cases resistant to therapy

WERNICKE-KORSAKOFF SYNDROME

- Wernicke's Encephalopathy - acute neurologic symptoms caused by thiamine deficiency
- Korsakoff's Psychosis -chronic neurologic symptoms caused by thiamine deficiency
- Treat with thiamine 500mg IV every 8 hours x 5 days

ENT

AURICULAR HEMATOMA

- Blunt trauma causes separation of perichondrium from underlying cartilage tears and their adjoining blood vessels
- Recurrent hematomas lead to infection and/or cartilage necrosis and cartilage formation (i.e. "cauliflower ear")
- Treatment requires drainage in the ENT after auricular block for anesthesia.
    - A compression dressing should be placed after drainage to prevent re-accumulation

EPISTAXIS

- >90% are anterior and occur along the nasal septum (kiesselbach plexus)
- <10% are posterior and occur from nasopalatine branch of sphenopalatine artery

Management consists of hemostatic control from

- **Direct nasal pressure**
- **Thrombogenic absorbable foams**
    - Gelfoam or Surgicel
- **Tranexamic acid**
    - 500mg TXA applied to topical foam or non absorbable packing and inserted into nares
- **Vasoconstrictive agents**
    - 0.05% oxymetazoline or phenylephrine
- **Chemical cautery**
    - Only perform unilaterally due to septal perforation risk
- **Anterior nasal packings**
    - Rapid Rhino
    - Merocel
    - Traditional Packing

- If nasal packing remains in place on discharge then prescribe a first generation cephalosporin or penicillin for prophylaxis against theoretical toxic shock syndrome
- Blood pressure control should not take priority over hemostatic control

EPIGLOTTITIS

- Strep, Staph, or H. flu mediated epiglottis infection
- May have the 3 D's: drooling, dysphagia, distress
- Lateral neck X-rays could show the "thumbprint sign"
- **Nebulized epinephrine can help decrease edema**
- Ceftriaxone 2gm IV once daily (first line) or
    - Cefotaxime 2gm (50mg/kg) IV three times daily or
    - Ampicillin/Sulbactam 3g (50mg/kg) IV q 6 hours or
    - Levofloxacin 750mg IV once daily
- Consider Vancomycin 15-20mg/kg to any of the above if risk of MRSA
- If immunocompromised: Cefepime 2g (50/kg) IV q8 hours and Vancomycin 15mg/kg IV q6 hours

LUDWIG'S ANGINA

- Bilateral infection of sub-mental, submandibular, and sublingual spaces
- Signs and Symptoms:
    - Dysphagia
    - Trismus
    - Edema of upper midline neck and floor of mouth
    - Raised tongue
    - "Woody" or brawny texture to floor of mouth with visible swelling and erythema
- Associated with IJ thrombophlebitis (Lemierre's Disease)
- Treatment must cover polymicrobial oral flora
- Most commonly a 3rd generation cephalosporin + (clindamycin or metronidazole)
- **If immunocompromised use cefepime + (clindamycin or metronidazole)**

OTITIS MEDIA

- Age 6mo - 2y: treat if there is otorrhea, severe symptoms, or bilateral involvement
- Age > 2y: treat if there is otorrhea or severe symptoms. Encourage a watch and wait prescription if no otorrhea and mild symptoms
- Amoxicillin 80-90mg/kg/day divided into 2 daily doses 7-10 days
- Amoxicillin/Clavulanate 80-90mg of amoxicillin per kg/day if treatment failure (prior 10 days)

OTITIS EXTERNA

- Floxin otic: 5 drops in affected ear BID x 7 days
    - Safe with perforations
- Cipro HC otic: 3 drops in affected ear BID x 7 days
    - Contains hydrocortisone therefore not safe with perforation
- CiproDex: 4 drops in affected ear BID x 7 days
    - Similar to Cipro HC but contains dexamethasone
- Cortisporin otic (neomycin/polymixin B/hydrocortisone)
    - 4 drops in ear TID-QID x 7days
    - Use suspension (NOT solution) if possibility of perforation

PERICHONDRITIS

- An infection of the connective tissue of the ear that covers the auricle or pinna
- Typically does not involve the lobule
- Cartilage is almost always involved with abscess formation and cavitation

Most common causes include minor trauma, burns, and ear piercing

May be a presenting symptom of immunosuppression

- HIV, Diabetes, Non-Hodgkin's lymphoma, or relapsing polychondritis
- Anti-Pseudomonas antibiotic therapy:
    - Ciprofloxacin 750mg q12 hours for 7 day or Clindamycin 450mg q6 hours for 7 days

MASTOIDITIS

- Inflammation of middle ear spreads into mastoid air cells
- Complications include, but are not limited to:
  - Meningitis/Encephalitis
  - Venous sinus thrombosis
  - Brain abscess
  - Facial nerve palsy
  - Sepsis
- CT with thin cuts through the mastoid with IV contrast provides diagnosis
- Coverage against S. pneumoniae, S. pyogenes, S. aureus, H. influenzae
  - Clindamycin 600mg IV q8 hours or (if MRSA concern use Vancomycin regimen)
  - Vancomycin 15-20mg/kg IV q12 hours and
  - Ceftriaxone 1g (50mg/kg) IV once daily or
  - Ampicillin/Sulbactam 3g (50mg/kg) IV q6 hours

TYMPANIC MEMBRANE TRAUMA

- Most tympanic perforations hear spontaneously
- Caution patient to avoid getting water behind the tympanic membrane

PERITONSILLAR ABSCESS

- Most common head and neck deep space infection
- Almost exclusively from Group A Strep infection
- Treat with Aspiration or I&D
- Antibiotics are only needed if aspiration is incomplete
  - Clindamycin 300mg PO Q6hrs x7-10d or
  - Amoxicillin/Clavulanate 875 mg PO BID x 7-10d or
  - Penicillin V 500mg PO + Metronidazole 500mg QID

RETROPHARYNGEAL ABSCESS

- Infection in the neck space anterior to the prevertebral fascia and posterior to the pharynx.
- Most common in children less than 5 years old

- Soft tissue neck X-ray may show a widened retropharyngeal space although CT neck with IV contrast is the gold standard
- The prevertebral space should be less than 7mm at C2, 14mm at C6 in children regardless of the age and 22mm at C6 in adults
- Requires surgical drainage by ENT.
    - Clindamycin 600-900mg IV or
    - Cefoxitin 2gm IV or
    - Ampicillin/Sulbactam 3g IV

PHARYNGITIS

Centor Criteria: one point for each of the criteria:

- Absence of a cough
- Swollen and tender cervical lymph nodes
- Temperature >38.0 °C (100.4 °F)
- Tonsillar exudate or swelling
- Age less than 15 (subtract a point if age >44)
- Probability os strep pharyngitis based on centor: (1 or less (10%), 2 (11-17%), 3 (28-35%), 4-5 (52%)
- Consider treatment if score is 4-5.

Penicillin treatment options

- Penicillin V 250mg PO BID x 10d (child) or 500mg BID x 10d (adolescent or adult)
- Bicillin L-A <27 kg: 0.6 million units; ≥27 kg: 1.2 million units IM x 1

Penicillin allergic treatment options

- Cefuroxime 10mg/kg PO QID x 10d (child) or 250mg PO BID x 4d or
- Clindamycin 7.5mg/kg PO QID x 10d (child) or 450mg PO TID x 10d or
- Azithromycin 12mg/kg QD (child) or 500mg on day 1; then 250mg on days 2-5
- **Consider single dose of dexamethasone 0.6mg/kg PO (Max = 10mg)**

DRY SOCKET

- Also known as Acute alveolar osteitis
- Caused by premature loss of healing clot in the alveolar socket after tooth extraction
- Occurs 2-4d after tooth extraction
- Initial post-extraction pain subsides followed by sudden/severe pain at extraction site

Treatment

- Analgesia (via apical dental block)
- Do not remove any residual clot
- Pack with iodoform ribbon gauze soaked with eugenol (oil of cloves) or local anesthetic
- Clindamycin 300mg PO Q8hrs x 5 days

PULPITIS

- Acute local tooth pain associated with cold or heat, sweat or sour food.
- For irreversible pain definitive care requires a root canal.
- Apical dental block can provide local analgesia in addition to irritant avoidance

PERIAPICAL ABSCESS

- Dental caries or nonviable teeth create a nidus for infection
- Local I&D can help relieve pan
- Antibiotics target to polymicrobial oral flora prevent subsequent worsening infections
    - Clindamycin 300mg PO q8 hours or
    - Ampicillin/Sulbactam 3g IV q6 hours

CAVERNOUS SINUS THROMBOSIS

- A complication of sinusitis or paranasal sinus infections that lead to a thrombus that extends extension to opposite sinus.
- Structures within the Cavernous Sinus can be all or partially affected
    - V1 and V2
    - III, IV, VI

- Internal Carotid Artery
- MRI+MRV are the imaging modalities of choice
- Clinical signs of fever, infraorbital/periorbital cellulitis, proptosis (uni/bl), decreased visual acuity, cranial nerve palsy secondary to CN III, IV, VI
- CN VI typically affected 1st causing lateral gaze palsy

ACUTE NECROTIZING ULCERATIVE GINGIVITIS

- Aka "Trench Mouth"
- Periodontal lesions, bacteria invade non-necrotic tissue

Uncomplicated Disease

- Amoxicillin/Clavulanate 875 mg PO two times daily and
    - Metronidazole 500mg PO three times daily x 7 days   or
- Clindamycin 300mg PO three times daily or
- Doxycycline 100 mg PO BID x 10 days

AIDS or immunocompromised increase the risk of candida infections

- Nystatin oral rinse four times daily x 14 days or
- Fluconazole 200mg PO daily x 14 days

ACUTE HEARING LOSS EVALUATION

- Most common cause is idiopathic although other causes include: viral (mumps), cerumen impaction, ototoxic medications, metabolic disturbances, and trauma

Weber test

- Place a vibrating tuning fork on the forehead, equidistant to both ears
- If the patient hears the sound equally in both ears, normal hearing or symmetric hearing loss is suspected.
- If sound is heard more in affected ear → consider conductive hearing loss in affected ear
- If sound is heard more in unaffected ear → consider sensorineural hearing loss in affected ear

Rinne test

- A vibrating turning fork is placed on the mastoid bone behind the ear. When the sound is no longer heard, the fork is held near the ear canal.
- If the sound is still present or louder at the ear canal, normal hearing is suspected. (i.e. Air conduction is greater than bone conduction)
- If no sound is heard near the ear canal but the sound was still heard on the mastoid bone, conductive hearing loss is suspected in that ear. (i.e. bone conduction > air conduction)

VESTIBULAR NEURITIS

- Self limiting cause of peripheral vertigo that should be distinguished from central vertigo
- Unlike labyrinthitis there should be no hearing loss (but symptoms may last up to 10 days)
- Symptomatically vertigo may require meclizine or low dose benzodiazepines

LABYRINTHITIS

- Infection of cochlear and vestibular apparatus (from middle ear via round/oval windows)
- Patients have peripheral vertigo + hearing loss + middle ear findings
- Suppurative form requires antibiotics (first gen. cephalosporin)
  - Prochlorperazine 10mg PO q6 PRN for nausea/vomiting
  - Lorazepam or diazepam as vestibular depressant

BENIGN PAROXYSMAL POSITIONAL VERTIGO

- Sudden-onset vertigo and associated nystagmus precipitated by head movements (often causing severe nausea and vomitting)
- Latency period <30s between provocative head position and onset of nystagmus
- Intensity of nystagmus increases to a peak before slowly resolving
- Duration of vertigo and nystagmus ranges from 5–40s (Paroxysm
- Repeated head positioning causes vertigo and nystagmus to fatigue and subside

- Nystagmus reverses direction during the head down and head up portions of Dix-Hallpike
- Nausea/vomiting common
- Symptoms worse in the morning (symptoms fatigue as day goes on)
- No associated hearing loss or tinnitus
- MUST distinguish from central vertigo

MÉNIÈRE'S DISEASE

- Occurs due to increased endolymph within the cochlea and labyrinth
- First attack usually occurs in patients >65yrs
- Usually is unilateral but may become bilateral with time
- No workup required for classical Ménière's disease in the ED Confirmed by ENT via glycerol testing or vestibular-evoked potentials
- Imaging with MRI if suspicion or need to rule out a central lesion

SIALOLITHIASIS

- Development of a calcium carbonate and calcium phosphate stone in a stagnant salivary duct
- >80% occur in the submandibular gland
- A stone may be palpated within the duct (most often unilateral)
- Treat with hydration, sialogogues (lemon candy) and in the rare cases ENT extraction

PAROTITIS

Viral parotitidis

- Paramyxoviruses (e.g. mumps), also from influenza, parainfluenza, coxsackie, echo, and acute HIV
- Most common in children <15yrs
- Self limited infections (except for HIV)

Suppurative parotitis

- Treatment targeted at S. aureus, gram negative bacilli, mumps, enteroviruses, and influenza virus
- Amoxicillin/Clavulanate 875mg (45mg/kg) PO BID or

- Clindamycin 450mg PO three times daily or 10mg/kg PO four times daily

SINUSITIS

- **Defined as 2 or more of the following:**
    - Blockage or congestion of nose
    - Facial pain or pressure
    - Hyposmia (diminished ability to smell)
    - Anterior or posterior nasal discharge lasting <12wk
- Rarely bacterial in origin, therefore rarely requiring antibiotics
- Likelihood of bacterial cause increases with the following
    - **Purulent discharge and pain on face or teeth > 10 days without improvement and**
    - Severe symptoms or fever > 39C plus symptoms > 3 days or
    - "Double sickening" - sinusitis symptoms at end of initially improving URI that lasted > 5 days

TRACHEITIS

- Most common in pediatric patients <10yo
- Patients will present with copious tracheal secretions, fever and stridor
- Soft tissue neck X-ray imaging is not required but may reveal subglottic tracheal narrowing
- Patients require antibiotics targeted to Staph. species and continued suctioning

ACUTE NECROTIZING ULCERATIVE GINGIVITIS (ANUG)

- Organisms involved are polymicrobial but often include Fusobacterium necrophorum, Treponema spp, and Prevotella

Immunocompetent

- Amoxicillin/Clavulanate 875 mg PO two times daily and
- Metronidazole 500mg PO three times daily x 7 days or

- Clindamycin 300mg PO three times daily or
  - Ciprofloxacin can substitute for Amoxicillin if patient is penicillin allergic.

Immunocompromised

- Patients have an increased risk of oral candida infection and should receive:
  - Nystatin oral rinse four times daily x 14 days or
  - Fluconazole 200mg PO daily x 14 days

Oral hygiene therapies

- Chlorhexidine 0.01% oral rinse BID or
- Magic Mouthwash (multiple variations) - 300cc of 1:1:1 viscous lidocaine 2%, Maalox, diphenhydramine 12.5mg/5ml elixir

EPIGLOTTITIS

- Coverage targets Streptococcus pneumoniae, Staphylococcus pyogenes, and Haemophilus influenzae, and Parainfluenza

Immunocompetent

- Ceftriaxone 2gm IV once daily (first line) or
- Cefotaxime 2gm (50mg/kg) IV three times daily or
- Ampicillin/Sulbactam 3g (50mg/kg) IV q 6 hours or
- Levofloxacin 750mg IV once daily

Immunocompromised

- Coverage should include the above regimen and coverage for Pseudomonas, M. tuberculosis, and MRSA
  - Cefepime 2g (50/kg) IV q8 hours and Vancomycin 15mg/kg IV q6 hours

DENTAL ABSCESS

- Treatment is broad and focused on polymicrobial infections and local antibiogram sensitivities
  - Penicillin VK 500mg PO q6 hours or
  - Clindamycin 300mg PO q8 hours or

- Ampicillin/Sulbactam 3g IV q6 hours

LUDWIG'S ANGINA

- Must cover typical polymicrobial oral flora and pseudomonas
  - Cefepime 2 g IV q12 hrs + Metronidazole 500 mg IV q6 hrs or
  - Meropenem 1 g IV q8 hrs or
  - Piperacillin-tazobactam 4.5g (80mg/kg) IV q6 hours
  - Add Vancomycin 15-20 mg/kg q8 hrs (max 2 g per dose) if concern for MRSA risk factors or immunocompromised

MASTOIDITIS

- Coverage against S. pneumoniae, S. pyogenes, S. aureus, H. influenzae
  - Clindamycin 600mg IV q8 hours or
  - Ceftriaxone 1g (50mg/kg) IV once daily or
  - Ampicillin/Sulbactam 3g (50mg/kg) IV q6 hours

OTITIS EXTERNA

- Floxin otic: 5 drops in affected ear BID x 7 days
  - Safe with perforations
- Cipro HC otic: 3 drops in affected ear BID x 7 days
  - Contains hydrocortisone to promote faster healing
  - Not safe with perforation
- Cortisporin otic (neomycin/polymixin B/hydrocortisone)
  - 4 drops in ear TID-QID x 7days
  - Use suspension (NOT solution) if possibility of perforation

STREPTOCOCCAL PHARYNGITIS

- Treatment can be delayed for up to 1 week and still prevent major sequelae (encouraging watch and wait prescriptions)
  - Penicillin V 250mg PO BID x 10d (child) or 500mg BID x 10d (adolescent or adult) or
  - Clindamycin 7.5mg/kg PO QID x 10d (child) or 450mg PO TID x 10d or

- Azithromycin 12mg/kg QD (child) or 500mg on day 1; then 250mg on days 2-5

PERITONSILLAR ABSCESS

- Coverage for Streptococcus species, anaerobes, Eikenella, H. influenza, S. aureus and requires definitive therapy with I&D

Outpatient Options

- Clindamycin 300mg PO Q6hrs x7-10d or
- Amoxicillin/Clavulanate 875 mg PO BID x 7-10d or
- Penicillin V 500mg PO + Metronidazole 500mg QID

Options if unable to take oral therapy

- Ampicillin/Sulbactam 3 gm (75mg/kg) IV four times daily or
- Piperacillin/Tazobactam 4.5 gm IV TID or
- Ticarcillin/Clavulanate 3.1 g IV QID or
- Clindamycin 600-900mg IV TID or
- Penicillin G 4 million units (50,000 units/kg) IV four times daily + Metronidazole 500mg IV three times daily

Gastrointestinal

APPENDICITIS

- **Psoas sign** - RLQ pain with extension of the right hip
- **Obturator sign** - RLQ pain on internal rotation of flexed right hip
- **Rovsing's sign** - Rebound RLQ pain on palpation of LLQ
- Clinical exam findings and likelihood of appendicitis (LR+ greater than 10 provide greatest utility for increasing the probability of a disease)

Finding	LR+	LR-
RLQ pain	7.3-8.4	0-0.28
Rigidity	3.76	0.82
Migration	3.18	0.50
Pain before vomiting	2.76	NA
Psoas sign	2.38	0.90
Fever	1.94	0.58
Rebound	1.1-6.3	0-0.86
Guarding	1.65-1.78	0-0.54
No similar pain previously	1.5	0.32
Anorexia	1.27	0.64
Nausea	0.69-1.2	0.70-0.84
Vomiting	0.92	1.12

- Ultrasound is the preferred initial diagnostic test although limitations involve body habitus
- CT scan should be reserved for the adult males with equivocal findings
- MRI idea for equivocal findings in pediatric patients and women (pregnant or non-pregnant)

BARIATRIC SURGERY COMPLICATIONS

- All bariatric surgery patients are at risk for:
    - DVT and PE
    - Pneumonia
    - UTI
    - Small Bowel Obstruction
    - Gastric perforation
    - Surgical site and intraabdominal infections

ROUX-EN-Y SPECIFIC COMPLICATIONS

Gastric pouch

- The remaining "stomach" may rupture if distended
    - The Jejunojejunostomy attached my leak
- Diagnosis X-ray may show a large gastric air bubble

Marginal Ulcers

- Occur at the Jejunojejunostomy due to acid secretion
    - Ulcer may perforate or cause upper GI bleed

Cholelithiasis

- Rare in the modern day since most patients have a cholecystectomy during the roux-en-y

Hernias

- Ventral hernias
- Internal hernias
    - Intermittent and may be difficult to detect via CT (requires PO contrast)
    - Suspected may require urgent surgical exploration lest patient has strangulated pathology

Dumping Syndrome

- Occurs when pylorus is either removed or bypassed, allowing hyperosmolar stomach chyme to "dump" into the small intestine.
- Hyperosmolality of food → fluid shifts into GI lumen → causing abdominal pain diarrhea and even syncope.

- Insulin response that leads to hypoglycemia 2-3 hours after meal
- Causes dizziness, fatigue, diaphoresis, weakness

GASTRIC BANDING

- All of the following complications require CT with oral and IV contrast

Stomal Obstruction

- Early complication, typically due to inclusion over excess perigastric fat vs tissue edema vs inappropriate sized band
- Present with nausea/vomiting and pain

Gastric insufflation port infection

- Associated with band erosion
- Requires replacement of port or band + IV antibiotics towards staph./strep species

Band Erosion

- Gastric band erodes through the gastric wall generally many months after surgery
- Treatment with band removal and perforation repair if present

Band Slippage and gastric prolapse

- Can occur anterior or posterior with gastric obstruction like symptoms
- Treatment requires emergent surgical repair

Esophageal dilatation

- Caused from partial obstruction due to band over-inflated leading to esophageal dilation
- Band deflation improves symptoms

Hiatus hernia

- Can often been seen on chest X-ray

SLEEVE GASTRECTOMY

- A portion of the stomach is removed along the greater curvature of stomach

- All bariatric surgery patients are at risk for:
  - DVT and PE
  - Pneumonia
  - UTI
  - Small Bowel Obstruction
  - Gastric perforation
  - Surgical site and intraabdominal infections

ROUX-EN-Y SPECIFIC COMPLICATIONS

Gastric pouch

- The remaining "stomach" may rupture if distended
  - The Jejunojejunostomy attached my leak
- Diagnosis X-ray may show a large gastric air bubble

Marginal Ulcers

- Occur at the Jejunojejunostomy due to acid secretion
  - Ulcer may perforate or cause upper GI bleed

Cholelithiasis

- Rare in the modern day since most patients have a cholecystectomy during the roux-en-y

Hernias

- Ventral hernias
- Internal hernias
  - Intermittent and may be difficult to detect via CT (requires PO contrast)
  - Suspected may require urgent surgical exploration lest patient has strangulated pathology

Dumping Syndrome

- Occurs when pylorus is either removed or bypassed, allowing hyperosmolar stomach chyme to "dump" into the small intestine.
- Hyperosmolality of food → fluid shifts into GI lumen → causing abdominal pain diarrhea and even syncope.

- Insulin response that leads to hypoglycemia 2-3 hours after meal
- Causes dizziness, fatigue, diaphoresis, weakness

GASTRIC BANDING

- All of the following complications require CT with oral and IV contrast

Stomal Obstruction

- Early complication, typically due to inclusion over excess perigastric fat vs tissue edema vs inappropriate sized band
- Present with nausea/vomiting and pain

Gastric insufflation port infection

- Associated with band erosion
- Requires replacement of port or band + IV antibiotics towards staph./ strep species

Band Erosion

- Gastric band erodes through the gastric wall generally many months after surgery
- Treatment with band removal and perforation repair if present

Band Slippage and gastric prolapse

- Can occur anterior or posterior with gastric obstruction like symptoms
- Treatment requires emergent surgical repair

Esophageal dilatation

- Caused from partial obstruction due to band over-inflated leading to esophageal dilation
- Band deflation improves symptoms

Hiatus hernia

- Can often been seen on chest X-ray

SLEEVE GASTRECTOMY

- A portion of the stomach is removed along the greater curvature of stomach

- Complication at any time include:
  - Bleeding at the staple line
- Stenosis causing gastric outlet obstruction
- Gastric leaks
- Treat of all conditions requires surgical repair

CIRRHOSIS COMPLICATIONS

- Ascites
- Esophageal varices
- Hepatic encephalopathy
- Spontaneous bacterial peritonitis
- Hepatorenal syndrome
- Portal hypertension
- Upper gastrointestinal bleed
- Hepatocellular carcinoma

ASCITES

Caused by

- Hepatitis or cirrhosis
- Heart failure or constrictive pericarditis
- Malignancy (primary or metastatic peritoneal carcinoma)
- Pancreatitis
- Vasculitis
- Connective tissue disorders
- Chylous ascites

Manage with

- Diuresis
- Optimization of renal fuction (spironolactone, diuretics, cardiac output optimization)
- Paracentesis if severe or possibility of an infection
- Water restriction

- Paracentesis

SPONTANEOUS BACTERIAL PERITONITIS

- Presence or abscess of abdominal pain cannot accurate predict the presence or absence of SBP. Diagnosis and rule out requires a paracentesis
- SBP rarely develops in patients without portal hypertension

Ascites fluid studies

- Cell count with differential
- Gram stain
- Culture (10cc in blood culture bottle)
- Glucose
- Protein

Diagnosis

- Absolute neutrophil count (PMNs) ≥250 or
- Bacteria on gram stain (single type)
- For bloody tap, subtract 1 WBC for every 250 RBC

Treatment

- 3rd-generation cephalosporin preferably:
- Cefotaxime 2g IV q8hr or Ceftriaxone 1-2g IV q12-24hr
- If allergic to above then, ciprofloxacin 400mg IV q12hr

If on peritoneal dialysis

- Cell count >100/mm with >50% neutrophils most consistent with infection
- Peritoneal dialysis associated SBP requires intraperitoneal antibiotics for Staphylococcus aureus or Staphylococcus epidermidis and Gram-negative enteric organisms.Infectious Diarrhea

Campylobacter jejuni

- Erythromycin 500mg PO BID x 5 days
- Ciprofloxacin 500mg PO BID x 5 days or
- Azithromycin 500mg PO once daily x 5 days

Entamoeba Histolytica

- Metronidazole 750mg PO three times daily for 5-10 days and
- Paromomycin 500mg q8hrs for 7 days or
- Iodoquinol 650mg q 8hrs daily 20 days

Giardia lamblia

- Metronidazole 250mg PO q8hrs for 7-10days

Microsporidium

- Albendazole 400mg PO BID x 21 days + HAART therapy if HIV positive

Salmonella

- TMP/SMX 1 DS tab PO BID x 5 days or
- Ceftriaxone 2g IV once daily x 5 days or
- Ciprofloxacin 500mg PO BID x 5 days

Shigella

- Ciprofloxacin 500mg PO BID x 5 days or
- TMP/SMX 1 DS tab PO BID x 5 days or
- Azithromycin 500mg PO daily x 5 days

Vibrio Cholerae

- Doxycycline 300mg PO as single dose or
- TMP/SMX 1 tablet (5mg/kg) PO BID daily x 3 daily

Yersinia enterocolitica

- Ciprofloxacin 500mg PO BID daily or
- TMP/SMX 1 DS tab (5mg/kg) PO BID

BLEEDING ESOPHAGEAL VARICES

Antibiotics

- For short-term prophylaxis against SBP and bacteremia

Other Medications

- Consider octreotide (50 mcg IV bolus, then 50 mcg/hr continuous, maintained at 2-5 days)
- Consider vasopressin 0.4 unit bolus, then infuse at 0.4 - 1 unit/min
- Pantoprazole or esomeprazole 80mg x 1; then 8mg/hr
- Intermittent dosing of pantoprazole, esomeprazole, or omeprazole 40 mg IV BID not inferior to continuous infusion dosing
- Reduces the rate of re-bleeding and need for surgery if there is an ulcer, but does not reduce morbidity or mortality

RPRBCl transfusion indications

- Hemoglobin <7 g/dl or hypotension
- In hemodynamically stable patients, the goal transfusion threshold should be 7 g/dl; NICE guidelines recommend avoidance of over-transfusion

Endoscopy

- Should be performed at the discretion of the gastroenterologist; within 12 hrs for variceal bleeding

HEPATIC ENCEPHALOPATHY

- Ammonia elevation due to accumulation of nitrogenous waste products normally metabolized by the liver
- Degree of hyperammonemia does not correlate with clinical symptoms
  - Stage I - General apathy
  - Stage II - Lethargy, drowsiness, variable orientation, asterixis
  - Stage III - Stupor with hyperreflexia, disorientation
  - Stage IV - Coma
- Treat with lactulose 20g PO or (300mL in 700cc H2O retention enema x30min)
  - In colon degrades into lactic acid: acidic environment traps ammonia
  - Also inhibits ammonia production in gut wall

HEPATORENAL SYNDROME

- Acute renal failure in patients with normal kidneys in the presence of acute or worsening chronic hepatic failure

- Emergent evaluation should focus on recognition and evaluation of acute electrolyte abnormalities, uremia, or hypervolemia
- Long term treatment involves optimizing hepatic function, protein status, and renal perfusion

ALCOHOLIC CIRRHOSIS

- Damage (irreversible) from chronic alcohol ingestion leading to hepatocytic nodules and fibrous tissue
- Porto-systemic shunting occurs due to portal hypertension leading to increased risk of developing
    - Abdominal ascites
    - Encephalopathy
    - Esophageal and rectal varices
    - Hepatorenal syndrome

ALCOHOLIC HEPATITIS

- Classic pattern involves AST > ALT elevation
- Chronic alcoholic hepatitis can manifest with
    - Macrocytic anemia
    - Elevated bilirubin and alkaline phosphatase
    - Thrombocytopenia can develop in the setting of portal hypertension

ALCOHOLIC STEATOSIS

- Liver capsule distention can cause acute or chronic right upper quadrant pain
- Generally no LFT derangement and pain is self limiting after alcohol cessation

UPPER GI BLEED

- Bleeding originating proximal to ligament of Treitz
- Risk Factors:
    - Medications
    - ASA, steroids, anticoagulants

- NSAIDs
- ETOH abuse
- Peptic ulcer disease, gastritis, varices
- Aortic graft (can cause aortoenteric fistula)

Initial Resuscitation

- Place 2 large bore IVs and monitor airway status
- Crystalloid IVF can be used for initial resuscitation but should be limited due to the dilutional anemia and dilatational coagulopathy that can result

Proton Pump Inhibitor

- Pantoprazole or esomeprazole 80mg x 1; then 8mg/hr
  - Intermittent dosing of pantoprazole, esomeprazole, or omeprazole 40 mg IV BID not inferior to continuous infusion dosing
  - Reduces the rate of re-bleeding and need for surgery if there is an ulcer, but does not reduce morbidity or mortality
  - There may be a mortality benefit in Asian patients

Antibiotics

- Ceftriaxone 1gm daily x 7 days (first line) or or ciprofloxacin IV or PO 500mg BID x7 days
- Should be administered as soon as possible in the ED
- For SBP and bacteremia prophylaxis for patients with confirmed or suspected variceal bleeding

Additional medication for consideration

- Octreotide (50 mcg IV bolus, then 50 mcg/hr continuous, maintained at 2-5 days)
- Vasopressin
  - 0.4 unit bolus, then infuse at 0.4 - 1 unit/min
  - Associated with many vasoconstrictive complications to include peripheral necrosis, dysrhythmias, myocardial ischemia
- Erythromycin 3mg/kg IV over 20-30min, 30-90min prior to endoscopy

Blood Transfusion

- Hemoglobin <7 g/dl in hemodynamically stable patients
- Any GI bleed patient that is hemodynamically unstable should receive and immediate blood transfusion as the hemoglobin value by lab can lag behind the actual value
- Evaluate for coagulopathy and correct with PCC or FFP

Balloon tamponade with Sengstaken-Blakemore Tube

- Reserved for life-threatening hemorrhage if endoscopy is not available

Endoscopy

- Ideally should be performed within 12 hours of bleeding

LOWER GI BLEED

- Distal to the ligament of Treitz
- Ealuate for coagulopathy
- IV fluids if needed for hemodynamic support
- Transfusion if hemoglobin < 7 mg/dL or unstable
- Emergent sigmoidoscopy/colonoscopy (next 24 hours)

FALSE POSITIVE FECAL OCCULT TEST

- Red meat
- Red jello
- Melon, broccoli, radish, beets
- Iron

ANAL FISSURES

- The majority are posterior midline
- Treat with stool softeners and sitz baths

ANAL FISTULAS

- **A connection from anal canal to the skin often caused by:**
  - Prior surgeries

- Prior or current infections
- Inflammatory bowel disease
- Malignancies
- Radiation Therapy

HEMORRHOIDS

- Engorgement of internal or external hemorrhoidal plexus which then becomes engorged, prolapsed, or thrombosed
- **Internal hemorrhoid**
  - Originate above the dentate line
  - Generally painless but may bleed
- **External hemorrhoid**
  - Originate below the dentate line
  - Painful if thrombosed
- Symptomatic treatment with topical anesthetics and stool softeners to minimize straining

TRACHEOESOPHAGEAL FISTULAS

- Manifests in pediatric patients due to a congenital deformity and presents with cyanosis or persistent coughing during feeds

CHOLECYSTITIS

- Most often isolated organisms are Escherichia coli, Klebsiella pneumonia, and anaerobes, especially Bacteroides fragilis
- Acute infection of the gallbladder usually in the setting of cholelithiasis but can be acalculous and requires emergent cholecystectomy
- Complications
  - **Emphysematous cholecystitis**
    - Due to secondary infection of GB by gas-forming organisms (C. perfringens)
  - **Mirizzi Syndrome**
    - Partial obstruction of common hepatic duct due to stone impaction / chronic inflammation
  - **Gallstone Ileus**

- Due to cholecystoenteric fistula
- **Gangrenous Cholecystitis**
    - Occurs in chronic untreated cholecystitis

CHOLANGITIS

- An infection of the biliary tract in the setting of cholelithiasis
- Charcot's Triad: Fever + jaundice + RUQ pain
- Reynold's Pentad: The triad + altered mental status + hypotension
- Coverage is targeted at E. coli, Enterococcus, Bacteroides, and Clostridium (anaerobic)
    - Metronidazole 500mg IV q8hrs and Ciprofloxacin 400mg IV q12hrs or
    - Piperacillin/Tazobactam 4.5g IV q8hrs or
    - Imipenem/Cilastin 500mg IV q6hrs or
    - Doripenem 500mg IV q8hrs or
    - Meropenem 1g IV q8hrs
    - Expand coverage for MRSA if severe sepsis or septic shock
        - Vancomycin 15-20mg/kg and any of the following options

INFLAMMATORY BOWEL DISEASE

- Treatment of an Acute flare requires, IV fluids if hypovolemic, bowel rest, analgesia, electrolyte correction, and consider a steroid burst in coordination with a GI consult
- **Inpatient admission if significant**
    - Metabolic derangements or profound hypovolemia with inability to tolerate hydration by mouth
    - Fulminate colitis
    - Obstruction
    - Peritonitis
    - Significant lower GI hemorrhage
- **Surgical consult if:**
    - Perforation
    - Abscess/fistula formation
    - Toxic megacolon

- **Chrons**
  - Can involve any part of the GI tract from the mouth to the anus
- **Ulcerative Colitis**
  - Inflammation tends to be progressively more severe from proximal to distal colon

DIVERTICULITIS

- Diverticular disease can be both left-sided colon (descending colon and sigmoid) or right-sided
- Stable patients with history of confirmed diverticulitis do not require further diagnostic evaluation
- 1st time episode or current episode different from previous requires diagnostic imaging (CT abd/pelvis with IV contrast)
- Antibiotics are aimed at treating Gram Negative organisms and Anaerobes
  - Metronidazole 500mg PO Q8hrs and Ciprofloxacin 500mg PO BID x10-14d or
  - Amoxicillin/Clavulanate 875/125 PO BID x10-14d or
  - Trimethoprim/Sulfamethoxazole, one double-strength tablet bid, and Metronidazole 500 mg Q8h

DYSPHAGIA

- Differential diagnosis is dependent on the phase of swallowing that is affected

Oropharyngeal dysphagia

- CVA
- Parkinson's disease
- Brain stem tumors
- Degenerative disease - ALS, MS, Huntington's
- Post-infectious - polio, syphilis
- Peripheral neuropathy
- Myasthenia gravis
- Polymyositis, dermatomyositis
- Muscular dystrophy

- Esophageal dysphagia

Achalasia

- Diffuse esophageal spasm
- Esophageal foreign body
- Esophageal web
- Malignancy, mediastinal masses
- Schatzki Ring
- Scleroderma
- Strictures - peptic, radiation, chemical, medication-induced
- Vascular compression
- Zenker's diverticulum

CHOLECYSTITIS

- Most often isolated organisms are Escherichia coli, Klebsiella pneumonia, and anaerobes, although definitive therapy is surgery
    - Metronidazole 500mg IV q8hrs and
    - Ciprofloxacin 400mg IV q12 hrs or
    - Levofloxacin 750mg IV q24hrs or
    - Ceftriaxone 1g IV q24hrs
- Add Vancomycin 15-20mg/kg if abscess or perforation

CLOSTRIDIUM DIFFICILE

- Vancomycin 125 mg PO (IV form ineffective) four times daily or
- Fidaxomicin 200 mg PO two times daily or
- Metronidazole 500mg PO or IV q6hr x10-14d (no longer first line)

DIVERTICULITIS

- Metronidazole 500mg PO Q8hrs and Ciprofloxacin 500mg PO BID x10-14d or
- Amoxicillin/Clavulanate 875/125 PO BID x10-14d or
- Trimethoprim/Sulfamethoxazole, one double-strength tablet bid, and Metronidazole 500 mg Q8h

PERITONEAL DIALYSIS ASSOCIATED PERITONITIS

Empiric Therapy (Intraperitoneal)

- Can be administered outpatient with coordination with nephrology:
    - Vancomycin 30mg/kg loading followed by 0.6 mg/kg IP daily and
    - Ceftazidime 1g IP daily or
    - Gentamycin 0.6mg/kg daily
- If arrangement of IP antibiotics is unfeasible then IV antibiotics can be considered

TRAVELER'S DIARRHEA

- Coverage targeted empirically towards E. coli, Campylobacter, Salmonella, and Shigella
    - Ciprofloxacin 750mg PO once daily x 1-3 days or
    - Azithromycin 500mg PO q24h x 3 days or 1000mg PO x 1

ESOPHAGEAL FOREIGN BODY

CXR PA and lateral

- Coins in esophagus present their face on AP view
- Coins in trachea present their face on lateral view
- Bones can only be visualized <50% of time
- Button batteries may present with "double-ring sign"

CT chest

- Very high-yield for both radiopaque and non-radiopaque objects but often not needed and generally avoided due to radiation risk for young patients
- Sensitivity >99% and specificity 70-92%

Indications for Urgent Endoscopy

- Complete obstruction of esophagus (pooling, risk of aspiration)
- Ingestion of button batteries
- Esophageal perforation
- Coin at the level of the cricopharyngeus muscle (C6) in children

BOERHAAVE SYNDROME

- Full thickness perforation of the esophagus
- Mackler's triad
- Pathognomonic for Boerhaave syndrome (chest pain, vomiting, subcutaneous emphysema)
- Chest x-ray or CT chest will make the diagnosis with the presence of pneumomediastinum

MALLORY WEISS TEAR

- Most Mallory-Weiss tears are minor and resolve on their own, but up to 3% of upper gastrointestinal bleeding deaths are a result of Mallory-Weiss tears
- Endoscopy only for active and on-going bleeding
- Most tears self resolve and just require outpatient supportive care

ESOPHAGITIS

- Causes include:
    - Corrosive ingestions
    - Radiation exposure
    - Pill ingestion
    - Infections
    - In immunocompromised patient always consider candida and try fluconazole

FOOD BOLUS IMPACTION

- Esophageal impaction can result in airway obstruction, stricture, or perforation. Perforation can be due to multiple mechanisms but is generally either mechanical (e.g. ingested bones) or via chemical corrosion (button battery)
- Uncomplicated food impaction (no bones, incomplete obstruction) can be managed expectantly
- Food bolus to remain impacted for >12-24hr. It is reasonable to consider therapies such as glucagon or a carbonated beverage
    - Glucagon 1-2mg IV/IM (adults) to relax LES - may cause severe nausea/vomiting

HERNIAS

- Irreducible hernias = incarcerated
- Can lead to vascular compromise if strangulated

MESENTERIC ISCHMIA

- Pain out of proportion to exam often paired with an elevated lactate
- Hypovolemic states require resuscitation while embolic and thrombotic related ischemia require anticoagulation and a surgical consult
- **Mesenteric arterial embolism**
    - Can be caused by dysrhythmias or valvular disease
- **Mesenteric arterial thrombosis**
    - Caused by hypercoagulable states or atherosclerosis
- **Mesenteric venous thrombosis**

- Caused by hypercoagulable states
- **Nonocclusive mesenteric ischemia**
  - Severe hypovolemic states + mesenteric arterial insufficiency

PANCREATITIS

Diagnosis requires either: characteristic abdominal pain or lipase level >3x upper limit of normal

Ranson's Criteria for Pancreatitis Mortality

Score of 3 or more indicates severe acute pancreatitis.

- **On admission**
  - Age > 55
  - WBC > 16,000
  - Blood glucose >200mg/dL
  - Lactate dehydrogenase >350 U/L
  - Aspartate aminotransferase (AST) >250 U/L
- **48 hours**
  - Hematocrit fall by > 10%
  - BUN increase by >5mg/dL
  - Serum Calcium <8mg/dL
  - pO2 < 60mmHg
  - Base deficit >4 mEq/L
  - Fluid Sequestration > 6L
- In addition to identifying the cause (hyperlipidemia, gallstones, drugs or envenomation) treatment should focus on fluid resuscitation, analgesia and pancreatic rest (NPO)

RECTAL PROLAPSE

- Circumferential protrusion of part or all layers of the rectum through the anal canal
- Reduction can generally be accomplished by applying pressure over the prolapsed mucosa and decreasing edema by applying an osmotic agent such as granulated sugar
- Failed reductions require emergent surgical consults due to the risk of ischemia

VOLVULUS

- In adults the majority of volvulus occur at the sigmoid in bedridden patients or those with chronic constipation.
- Abdominal X-ray or CT will show dilated loops of bowel at the volvulus site
- Requires surgical reduction

Hematology

COAGULOPATHY

Platelet Related

- Thrombocytopenia
- Nonfunctional
- Aspirin
- Von Willebrand disease

Clotting Factor Related

- Acquired (Drug Related)
- Warfarin (Coumadin)
- Heparinization
- Vitamin K deficiency
- Disseminated Intravascular Coagulation (DIC)
- Decreased factor production (liver disease)
- Uremic bleeding syndrome
- Hemophilia
- Factor VIII inhibitor
- Lupus anticoagulant

CRYOPRECIPITATE

- Cold insoluble protein fraction of FFP
- Contains: fibrinogen, vWF, and factor VIII
- 1 bag (10ml) has 50-500 units of factor 8 activity
- Indicated for
    - Bleeding with fibrinogen level of <100 milligrams/dL
    - Dysfibrinogenemia
    - Bleeding in vWD (in addition to DDAVP + Factor VIII repletion)

DDAVP (DESMOPRESSIN)

- Synthetic replacement for vasopressin and often given for Hemophilia A & Von Willebrand Disease
- IV: 0.3 mcg/kg IV over 15-30 minutes IV (for pre-op 30 min before procedure)
- intranasal:
    - <50 kg: 150 mcg; for pre-op, give 2 hr before procedure
    - >50 kg: 300 mcg; for pre-op, give 2 hr before procedure

HUMATE-P

- Human Plasma-derived von Willebrand Factor
- Contains both vWF and factor VIII
- Indicated for bleeding patients with Von Willebrand disease (use in conjunction with DDAVP

FRESH FROZEN PLASMA

- 1 bag = 1 unit = 250 mL
- 10-20 mL/kg (4-6 units in 70kg adult) will increase factors by ~20-30%
- Transfuse at least 15 mL/kg at a time (4 units in 70-kg adult)
- Contains all coagulation factors and fibrinogen
    - 40 mL/kg raises any factor by 100% (each unit is ~200mL)
- May cause fluid overload
- ABO compatibility a must but crossmatch before transfusing not
- INR of FFP is ~1.6; therefore transfusing for INR <1.7 is not advised

PLATELETS

- **Leukocyte reduced:** prevents sensitization in patients who may require bone marrow transplant
- **Irradiated**: eliminates capacity of T-cells to proliferate (prevents Transfusion-associated graft-versus-host disease)

Platelet transfusion thresholds

- <50K if planned lumbar puncture or neurosurgical procedure
- <20K if planned for central venous catheter placement (preference toward compressible site), or febrile patient

- <10K in asymptomatic patients (unless due to ITP, TTP, or HIT)
- Transfusion should be type specific because platelets are bathed in plasma

	ITP	TTP	HUS	HIT	DIC
Decreased platelets	Yes	Yes	Yes	Yes	Yes
Increased INR	No	No	No	-	Yes
MAHA	No	Yes	Yes	No	Yes
Low Fibrinogen level	No	No	No	No	Yes
Platelet transfusion is safe	Yes	No	No	No	Yes

PACKED RED BLOOD CELLS

- One unit (250mL) raises hemoglobin by 1 g/dl
- Pediatric dosing: 15 mL/kg.
- **Leukocyte reduced: Prevents sensitization in patients who may require bone marrow transplant**
- **Irradiated: Eliminates capacity of T-cells to proliferate (prevents transfusion-associated graft-versus-host disease)**

PROTHROMBIN COMPLEX CONCENTRATE

- 3 factor PCC (Factors II, IX, and X), would need to supplement with factor VII for reversal if using 3 factor PCC
- 4 factor PCC (Factors II, VII, IX, and X)
  - INR 2-4: 25units/kg, not to exceed 2500 units
  - INR 4-6: 35units/kg, not to exceed 3500 units
  - INR >6: 50units/kg, not to exceed 5000 units
- Consider rechecking INR after 15 minutes to determine need for redosing

THROMBOCYTOPENIA

- Thrombocytopenia is defined as platelets of less than 150 x 103/mcL. Symptoms such as bruising and petechiae usually occur at counts at 50 x 103/mcL and between 5-10x 103/mcL there is a high risk of spontaneous bleeding
- Decreased production

- Increased platelet destruction or use
- Drug Induced

TRANEXAMIC ACID

- Indicated for severely bleeding trauma patient, systolic blood pressure of <90 and/or heart rate > 110 beats/min, with expected requirement for massive transfusion.
- Total of 2 Grams
    - Initial bolus of 1 Gm over 10 minutes (Slow IV push).
    - Maintenance: additional 1 Gm over next 8 hours (mix in 50 mL of NS). Call Pharmacy to mix and deliver the continuous infusion

TRANSFUSION-RELATED ACUTE LUNG INJURY (TRALI)

- Acute onset hypoxemic respiratory failure due to non-cardiogenic pulmonary edema occurring during or shortly after transfusion
- Leads to inflammatory pulmonary edema

DISSEMINATED INTRAVASCULAR COAGULATION

- Bleeding or thrombosis can predominate although bleeding is more common
- Formation of fibrin within the circulation or fibrinolysis depletes clotting factors leading to organ failure

MAHA (MICROANGIOPATHIC HEMOLYTIC ANEMIA)

All of the following conditions can cause MAHA

- Disseminated Intravascular Coagulation (DIC)
- Thrombotic Thrombocytopenic Purpura (TTP)
- Hemolytic Uremic Syndrome (HUS)
- HELLP syndrome
- Heparin-Induced Thrombocytopenia (HIT)
- Hereditary spherocytosis
- Paroxysmal nocturnal hemoglobinuria (PNH)

- Malignant hypertension
- Scleroderma
- Antiphospholipid Syndrome (APS)

SICKLE CELL DISEASE

- Vaso-Occlusive Crisis
- Bony infarction
- Dactylitis
- Avascular necrosis of femoral head
- Gallbladder disease (stones)
- Respiratory distress and Chest pain
- Bacteria(especially salmonella)

HEMOPHILIA

- **Bleeding complications for all hemophilia types include:**
    - Hemarthroses
    - Hematomas
    - Mucosal bleeding
    - Intracranial bleeding
    - Hematurea
- Unless the patient knows their factor level assume a baseline of 0% and target factor repletion to a goal of 100% activity based on the formulas below

Hemophilia A

- Lack factor 8
- **Dose of Factor VIII = weight (kg) x % increased desired x 0.5**
- **1 IU/kg will increase the plasma concentration by 2%**

Hemophilia B

- Lack factor 9
- **Dose of Factor IX = weight (kg) x % increase desired**
- **1 IU/kg will increase the plasma concentration by 1%**

VWD

- Most common inherited bleeding disorder
- **vWF has two roles:**
  - Acts as cofactor for platelet adhesion
  - Acts as carrier protein for factor VIII extending its half life
- VWF and factor VIII concentration is the first line therapy for vWD bleeding patients (combination therapy is found in Humate-P.
- Similar to hemophilia repletion, target 50 IU/kg for any major bleeding

HENOCH SCHONLEIN PURPURA (HSP)

- Most common childhood vasculitis
- Associated with an increased intussusception risk

Triad of

- **Non-thrombocytopenic palpable purpura**
- **Abdominal pain**
- **Arthritis**

THROMBOCYTOPENIA

Decreased production

- Marrow infiltration (tumor or infection)
- Viral infections (rubella, HIV)
- Marrow Suppression (commonly chemotherapy or radiation)
- Congentital thrombocytopenia
- Fanconi anemia
- Alport syndrome
- Bernand Soulier
- Vitamin B12 and/or folate deficiency

Increased platelet destruction or use

- Idiopathic thrombocytopenic purpura
- Thrombotic Thrombocytopenic Purpura (TTP)
- Hemolytic Uremic Syndrome (HUS)
- Disseminated Intravascular Coagulation (DIC)
- Viral infections (HIV, mumps, varicella, EBV)

- Drugs (heparin, protamine)
- Postransfusion or Posttransplantation
- Autoimmune destruction (SLE or Sarcoidosis)
- Mechanical destruction
- Artificial valves
- ECMO
- HELLP syndrome
- Excessive hemorrhage
- Hemodialysis, extracorporeal circulation
- Splenic Sequestration

Drug Induced

ONCOLOGIC EMERGENCIES

Related to Local Tumor Effects

- Malignant airway obstruction
- Bone metastases and pathologic fractures
- Malignant spinal cord compression
- Malignant Pericardial Effusion and Tamponade
- Superior vena cava syndrome

Related to Biochemical Derangement

- Hypercalcemia of malignancy
- Hyponatremia due to SIADH
- Adrenal insufficiency
- Tumor lysis syndrome
- Carcinoid syndrome

Related to Hematologic Derangement

- Neutropenic fever
- Neutropenic enterocolitis (typhlitis)
- Leukostasis and hyperleukocytosis
- Hyper-viscosity syndrome
- Thromboembolism

Related to Therapy

- Chemotherapy-induced nausea and vomiting
- Chemotherapeutic drug extravasation
- Differentiation syndrome (retinoic acid syndrome) in APML
- Stem cell transplant complications
- Catheter-related complications
- Tunnel infection
- Exit site infection
- CVC obstruction (intraluminal or catheter tip thrombosis)
- Catheter-related venous thrombosis
- Fracture of catheter lumen

IMMUNE THROMBOCYTOPENIC PURPURA (ITP)

- The disease follows a course that is usually stable with intermittent and episodic flares, leading to clinically relevant thrombocytopenia. Treatment options are:
- Corticosteroids - first line for adult patients
- Intravenous Immunoglobulin G (IVIG) 1gm/kg/d x 2 days - first line for adult patients
- Platelet transfusion - Indicated for life-threatening bleeding since platelets will ultimately be destroyed

HYPER-VISCOSITY SYNDROME

- Increased serum viscosity due to:
- Increased blood products (polycythemia, thrombocytosis, leukemia)
- Immunoglobulins (Waldenstrom's, IgA myeloma, multiple myeloma)
- Symptoms arise from poor capillary flow and organ congestion
- Provide viscosity dilution with IC fluids and either:
    - Leukopheresis - Leukostasis
    - Plateletpheresis - Thrombocytosis
    - Phlebotomy - Polycythemia

TRANSPLANT COMPLICATIONS

- Infection (39%)
- Noninfectious GI/GU pathology (15%)
- Dehydration (15%)
- Electrolyte disturbances (10%)
- Cardiopulmonary pathology (10%)
- Injury (8%)
- Rejection (6%)
- Acute graft-versus-host disease occurs in 20% to 80% of patients post-hematopoietic stem cell transplantation (HSCT); rarely occurs in solid organ transplant

TUMOR LYSIS SYNDROME

- Associated with treatment of ALL, Burkitt lymphoma, NHL
- Rarely observed in solid tumors or without prior therapy
- Rapid turnover of tumor cells (spontaneously or after treatment) leading to release of:
    - **Potassium**
    - **Phosphate**
    - **Binds Ca causing hypocalcemia**
    - **Uric acid (converted from nucleic acids)**
- Treat with aggressive hydration (1-2 ml/kg/hr of urine output) and each electrolyte abnormality

Infectious Disease

CMV RETINITIS

Severe Vision Threatening

- Ganciclovir intraocular implant for 8 months and
- Valganciclovir 900mg PO q12hrs x 14 days FOLLOWED BY 900mg PO q24hrs x 7 days

Peripheral lesions

- Valganciclovir 900mg PO q12hrs x 21 days FOLLOWED BY 900mg PO q24hrs x 7 days

CMV ESOPHAGITIS, COLITIS, OR NEUROLOGIC DISEASE

- Ganciclovir 5mg/kg IV q12hrs daily x 21 days (or until symptom resolution)
- Foscarnet 90mg/kg IV q12 hrs daily x 21 days (or until symptom resolution)

CMV PNEUMONIA

- Ganciclovir 5mg/kg IV q12hrs x 3 weeks
- Cryptococcosis
- Pulmonary (not AIDs associated)
- Fluconazole 400mg PO IV q24hrs x 6-12 months or
- Itraconazole 200mg PO q12hrs daily x 6-12 months or
- Voriconazole 200mg PO q12hrs x 6-12 months

Pulmonary (with AIDS)

- Fluconazole 400mg PO q24hrs x 6-12 months
- Meningitis (not AIDs associated)
- Amphotericin B 0.7-1mg/kg IV q24hrs and Flucytosine 25mg/kg PO q6hrs x 4 weeks
- Followed by Fluconazole 400mg PO q24hrs x 8 weeks

Meningitis (with AIDS)

- Amphotericin B 0.7-1mg/kg IV q24hrs and Flucytosine 25mg/kg PO q6hrs x 2 weeks
- Followed by Fluconazole 400mg PO q24hrs x 8 weeks
- Initiation of HAART is delayed by 2 to 10 weeks to minimize the risk of immune reconstitution syndrome

PNEUMOCYSTIS PNEUMONIA (PCP)

- TMP/SMX 2 DS tablets PO q8hrs daily or
- Dapsone 100mg PO once daily and TMP 5mg/kg PO q8hrs or
- Primaquine 30mg PO q24hrs and Clindamycin 450mg PO q8hrs

Prophylaxis

- TMP/SMX 1 double strength tablet daily, but one single strength tablet daily or one double-strength three times weekly is acceptable.

TOXOPLASMOSIS

Immunocompetent

- Pyrimethamine 200mg PO one dose (for loading) THEN 50mg PO q24hrs x4wks and
- Leucovorin 10mg PO q24hrs and
- Sulfadiazine 1g PO q6hrs

Immunocompromised

- TMP/SMX 5mg/kg IV q12hrs or
- Pyrimethamine 200mg PO one dose (for loading) THEN 75mg PO q24hrs x4-8wks and Leucovorin 25mg PO q24hrs and
- Sulfadiazine 1500mg PO q6hrs or

NEISSERIA MENINGITIDIS

Prophylaxis regimen

- Ciprofloxacin 500mg PO x1 or

- Rifampin 600mg PO BID x2d or
- Ceftriaxone 250mg IM x1

LYMPHOGRANULOMA VENEREUM

- Doxycycline 100mg PO BID x 21 days (first choice) or
- Erythromycin 500mg PO QID x 21 days or

SYPHILIS

Early

- Treatment Options:
- Penicillin G Benzathine 2.4 million units IM x 1
- Repeat dose after 7 days for pregnant patients and HIV infection
- Doxycycline 100mg oral twice daily for 14 days as alternative

Late Stage

- Late stage is greater than one year duration, presence of gummas, or cardiovascular disease
- Treatment Options:
- Penicillin G Benzathine 2.4 million units IM weekly x 3 weeks
- Doxycycline 100mg oral twice daily for 4 weeks as alternative

Neurosyphilis

- There are 3 Major options with none showing greater efficacy than others:
- Penicillin G 3-4 million units IV every 4 hours x 10-14 days
- Penicillin G 24 million units IV infusion 10-14 days
- Penicillin G Procaine2.4 million units IM daily + probenecid 500mg oral every 6 hours for 10-14 days.
- Alternative:
- Ceftriaxone 2gm IV once daily for 10-14 days
- Desensitization to the penicillin allergy is still the preferred method of treatment for patients with early and late stage disease (especially during pregnancy)

Pregnancy

- Penicillin, dosage depends on stage

NEUTROPENIC FEVER

- ANC <500 andFever ≥ 38.3°C (100.9°F)
- ANC = (total WBC) x (%segs + %bands)
- Nadir usually occurs by day 14 after chemotherapy
- **Antibiotic therapy should treat gram negative, gram positive, and pseudomonas and Mono-antibiotic appears to be as good as dual-drug therapy**
  - Cefepime 2g IV q8hr or Ceftazidime 2g IV q8hr OR
  - Imipenem/Cilastin 1gm IV q8hr or Meropenem 1gm IV q8hr OR
  - Piperacillin/Tazobactam 4.5gm IV q 6hr
- **Add vancomycin to above regimen for:**
  - Severe mucositis or MRSA colonization
  - Signs of catheter site infection or indwelling line
  - Hypotension

The MASCC risk Index can help score low-risk patients who can have close outpatient followup.

NEISSERIA MENINGITIDIS PROPHYLAXIS

- Ceftriaxone 250mg IM once (if less than 15yr then 125mg IM) or
- Ciprofloxacin 500mg PO once or
- Rifampin 600 mg PO BID x 2 days

HIV POST EXPOSURE PROPHYLAXIS

Superficial wound or solid needle

- If HIV+ source asymptomatic or if viral load <15000 RNA/mL give basic regimen
- If HIV+ with AIDS, acute seroconversion or high viral load give expanded regimen
- If HIV status unknown then no PEP (consider PEP if possible HIV risk from source)

Deep wound or hollow needle

- If HIV+ source asymptomatic or if viral load <15000 RNA/mL give expanded regimen
- If HIV+ with AIDS, acute seroconversion or high viral load give expanded regimen
- If HIV status unknown then no PEP (consider PEP if possible HIV risk from source)

Mucous Membrane Exposure

- If HIV+ source asymptomatic or if viral load <15000 RNA/mL consider basic regimen
- If HIV+ with AIDS, acute seroconversion or high viral load give basic regimen
- If HIV status unknown then no PEP (consider PEP if possible HIV risk from source)

HEPATITIS B POST-EXPOSURE PROPHYLAXIS

- Treatment is generally initiated after coordination with occupational health and infectious disease service and based the the exposed patient's vaccination history

Unvaccinated

- If the source is HBsAg(+) then give HBIG x1 and initiate HBV vaccine in two separate sites
- If source is HGsAG(-) then start the HBV vaccine series
- If source blood is unavailable and high risk then give HBIG x1 initiate the HBV series
- If source blood is low risk and unavailable then begin HBV series

Previously vaccinated non responder (one series)

- Non responder status is defined as anti-has <10mIU/mL
- If the source is HBsAg(+) then give HBIG x 1 and begin revaccination series
- Can also opt to perform second HBIG administration in one month
- If source is HBsAg(-) then no treatment is needed
- If source blood is unavailable and high risk then treat as if HBsAg(+)

Previously vaccinated non responder (two series)

- Non responder status is defined as anti-has <10mIU/mL
- If the source is HBsAg(+) then give HBIG x2 and no HBV series
- If source is HGsAG(-) then no treatment is needed
- If source blood is unavailable then initiate the HBV series

ENDOCARDITIS

- Diagnosis based on the Modified Duke Criteria

Dental procedure prophylaxis

- Generally not recommended except for patients with prosthetic valves or prior endocarditis
  - Clindamycin 600mg (20mg/kg) PO or
  - Amoxicillin 2g or 50mg/kg

Risk Factors

- IV Drug use (most often effecting the tricuspid valve)
- Prosthetic heart valve
- Rheumatic heart disease
- Mitral valve prolapse
- Bicuspid aortic valve
- Chronic indwelling lines
- Immunocompromised (HIV, chemotherapy)

Antibiotics for patients with native valves

- Ampicillin/Sulbactam 12g/day IV in 4 doses + Gentamicin 3mg/kg/day IV in 2 or 3 doses or
- Amoxicillin/Clavulanate 12g/day in 4 dose + Gentamicin 3mg/kg/day IV in 2 or 3 doses or
- Oxacillin or Nafcillin 2g IV six times daily + Gentamicin 1mg/kg IV three times daily AND Ampicillin 2g IV six times daily or
- Daptomycin 6mg/kg IV once daily

Antibiotics for patients with prosthetic valves

- Vancomycin 30mg/kg/day IV in 2 doses and
- Gentamicin 3mg/kg/day IV in 2 or 3 doses and

- Rifampin 1200 mg/day PO in 2 doses

SYPHILIS

- Primary lesions (chancre) appears after an 2-4 weeks of incubation
- Secondary rashes are often macular and non-pruritic but do not necessary start with the classic palms distribution.
- Rapid Plasma Reagin (RPR) is the ideal serum initial screening test while VDRL should be sent from CSF sample if neurosyphilis is suspected

Early syphilis includes primary, secondary, and early latent (less than one year)

- Penicillin G Benzathine 2.4 million units IM x 1 or
- Doxycycline 100mg oral twice daily for 14 days if PCN allergic

Late syphilis (> 1 year) involves gummas, aortitis, or cardiovascular disease

- Penicillin G Benzathine 2.4 million units IM weekly x 3 weeks or
- Doxycycline 100mg oral twice daily for 4 weeks if PCN allergic

Neurosyphilis

- Penicillin G 3-4 million units IV every 4 hours x 10-14 days or
- Penicillin G 24 million units continuous IV infusion 10-14 days or
- Ceftriaxone 2gm IV once daily for 10-14 days if PCN allergic

BOTULISM

- Clostridium botulinum produces toxin that blocks Ach release from presynaptic membrane
  - Horse derive antitoxin can be acquired from the CDC and health department
- Infantile botulism involves consumption of botulinum spores (honey, poorly stored food)
  - Requires treatment with Human-based Botulism IG (BabyBIG)
- **Patients present with symmetrical descending weakness leading to flaccid paralysis**

- Also can have anticholinergic signs
  - Decreased salivation
  - Urinary retention
  - Hyperthermia
  - Dilated pupils (in contrast to patients with myasthenia gravis)

PNEUMONIA (PEDS)

Newborn

- Hospitalized
- Ampicillin (80-90mg/kg/day) + gentamicin and/or cefotaxime
- Add vancomycin if MRSA a concern
- Add erythromycin (12.g mg/kg QID) if concern for chlamydia
- Outpatient
- Initial outpatient management not recommended

1-3 Month

- Hospitalized
- Afebrile pneumonitis
- Erythromycin (10 mg/kg q6) or azithro (2.5 mg/kg q12)
- Febrile pneumonia
- Add cefoTAXime (200mg/kg per day divided q8h)
- Outpatient
- erythromycin or azithro PO

>3mo - 18 years

- Hospitalized (PICU/severely ill)
- Ceftriaxone IV and vancomycin and consider azithromycin
- Hospitalized (moderately ill)
- Fully immunized: Ampicillin (50mg/kg q6) IV
- Not fully immunized: Ceftriaxone IV
- Outpatient
- Amoxicillin (90 mg/kg divided BID) x 5 days PO
- Alternative: clindamycin or azithromycin or amoxicillin-clavulanate

LICE

- Permethrin 1% lotion shampoo (if >2 months old)
- Wash hair with non-conditioned shampoo
- Apply Permethrin for 10 min and rinse

Eyelash Infestation

- Apply ophthalmic petroleum jelly q12hrs x 10 days
- Pediatrics <2yo
- Wet combing is an alternative to medical therapy

PINWORM

- Treatment targeted against Enterobius vermicularis
- Mebendazole 100mg PO once THEN repeat in 2 weeks or
- Albendazole 400mg PO once (100mig if < 2yo) THEN repeat in 2 weeks or
- Pyrantel Pamoate (Pin-x) 11mg/kg (max 1g) THEN repeat in 2 weeks

SCABIES

Adults

- Permethrin 5% cream for all family members
- Apply from neck dow and leave on for 8-12hr before washing off
- Ivermectin 200 mcg/kg may be necessary for severe infection
- Contraindicated in lactating women and children < 15kg

Infants

- Permethrin 5% is FDA approved for > 2 months of age although still recommended for neonatal scabies
- May require application head to toe (avoid mucus membranes) and leave on for 8-12 hours, then wash off

BABESIOSIS

- Each regimen is for 10 days duration and option 1 is often used for mild parasitemia <4% with option two for sever cases with >4% parasite load

- Atovaquone (750mg BID) and Azithromycin (500-1000mg on first day, 250-1000mg on subsequent days) or
- Clindamycin 600 mg PO q8h x 7-10 days

EHRLICHIOSIS

- Adults: Doxycycline 100mg PO/IV BID x 14 days
- Pediatrics: under 45 kg use Doxycycline 2.2mg/kg PO/IV twice a day
- Pregnant: Rifampin 300mg PO every 12 hours

MALARIA

- For non-pregnant patients (3 day course)
    - Artemether + lumefantrine
    - Artesunate + amodiaquine
    - Artesunate + mefloquine
    - Dihydroartemisinin + piperaquine
    - Artesunate + sulfadoxine–pyrimethamine (SP)

For pregnant (1st trimester)

    - Quinine + clindamycin x 7 days

Severe Malaria

- Do not delay treatment in the unstable patient if strong suspicion for malaria as initial smear may be falsely negative
    - Treatment (IV for ≥24 hours then 3 days PO course)
    - Artesunate (IV)
    - Clears malaria faster than quinine
    - Distributed only through CDC
    - Quinidine (IV) also appropriate choice; more available in US

TETANUS (ACUTE)

- Metronidazole 500mg IV (7.5mg/kg) q6hrs or
- Clindamycin 600mg IV (7.5mg/kg) q6hrs
- Penicillin

- Although once the drug of choice it is now no longer recommended since it may potentiate the effect of tetanus toxin by inhibiting the GABA receptors

PERTUSSIS

- Antibiotics do not help with severity or duration but may decrease infectivity.
- A reasonable guideline is to treat persons aged >1 year within 3 weeks of cough onset and infants aged <1 year and pregnant women (especially near term) within 6 weeks of cough onset.
- TMP--SMZ should not be administered to pregnant women, nursing mothers, or infants aged <2 months.
- The following regimens are for active disease or post-exposure prophylaxis. If a patient is has confirmed disease and is likely to be in contact with infants or pregnant women then the patient should be treated as up to 6-8 weeks after the onset of their illness.

< 1 month old

- Same antibiotics for active disease and post-exposure prophylaxis
- Azithromycin 10mg/kg (max 500mg/day) daily x 5 days

>1 month old

- Azithromycin 10mg/kg (max 500mg/day) daily x 5 days
- if > 6 months old then day 2-5 of treatment should be reduced to 5mg/kg (250mg/day max)
- TMP/SMX 4mg/kg PO BID daily for 14 days (if > 2 months old)

Adults

- Any of the following antibiotics are acceptable although azithromycin is most commonly prescribed
- Azithromycin 500mg PO once daily for day #1 then 250mg PO once daily for days #2-5
- Clarithromycin 500mg BID x7 days
- Erythromycin 500mg QID x7 days

BIOLOGIC IMMUNOMODULATORS

- Immunomodulators created by a mouse or human cell that either create antibodies or targets against various cell lines that are receptor based. They interact with cellular immunity such as tumor necrosis factor alpha and interleukins.
- The agent's uses range from a wide array of indications such as Crohn's disease, Ulcerative colitis and Inflammatory bowel disease, Rheumatoid arthritis, Psoriatic arthritis, Ankylosing spondylitis and many malignancies with specific receptors.
- The various letters chosen in the name indicated the structure, origin, and targets of the molecule. For example ixekizumab for psoriasis ends with –mab, so it is a monoclonal antibody, has a –u- so it is human and has –ki- which means that it is interleukin targeted.

Naming

- The various letters chosen in the name indicated the structure, origin, and targets of the molecule.
- For example ixekizumab for psoriasis ends with –mab, so it is a monoclonal antibody, has a –u- so it is human and has –ki- which means that it is interleukin targeted.

Suffix

- **-mab** means a monoclonal antibody
- **–cept** indicates a protein that mimics an immunoglobulin.

Middle syllable

- **–u-** means all human derived
- **-o-** means all mouse derived
- **-zu-** means humanized after being mouse derived
- **–xi-** means part-human and part-non human.

Middle bridging syllable

This lettering can indicate the biologic's target

- **t-** means tumor is the target.
- **–ba-** means there is bacterium target.
- **-so-** means bone is targeted.
- **–ci-** targets circulation.
- **–fu-** targets fungus.

- **–gro-** targets growth factor.
- **–ki- or –li-** which means it is interleukin or immune targeted.

Adverse events

- **Decreased cellular immunity which an cause reactivation or new:**
    - Tuberculosis
    - Sepsis
    - Fungal infections
    - Hepatitis B
- **Neurologic syndromes**
    - Multiple sclerosis
    - Seizures
    - Guillain-Barre syndrome
- **Hematologic side effects**
    - Aplastic anemia
    - Pancytopenia
- **Cardiac effects**
    - Congestive heart failure
    - Arrhythmias
- **Allergic reactions**
- **Pulmonary**
    - Pneumonia
    - Pneumocystis jirovecii pneumonia
    - Pneumonitis
- **Endocrine**
    - Thyroiditis
- **GI**
    - Perforations
    - Clostridium difficile
    - Acute bacterial infections
- **Malignancies**
    - Non-melanoma skin cancers
    - Lymphoma

Miscellaneous

ANAPHYLAXIS

- Type I hypersensitivity reaction that is either severe in nature or having two or more organ systems involved:
    - 'Cutaneous symptoms: Hives
    - Respiratory symptoms: Wheezing/Shortness of breath
    - Gastrointestinal symptoms: Diarrhea
    - Cardiovascular symptoms: Hypotension
- Biphasic reactions are rare and can occur anywhere from 10 minutes up to six days after an initial reaction
- **Treat with epinephrine 1:1000 IM 0.3 - 0.5mg (0.1mg/kg) every 5 - 15 minutes**

ANGIOEDEMA

- Angioedema is paroxysmal and rapid swelling of dermal or submucosal layers of skin or mucosa that is often asymmetric and non-pruritic.
- Icatibant: Bradykinin receptor antagonist
- Ecallantide: Kallikrein inhibitor

Allergic

- IgE–mediated type I hypersensitivity reaction
- Consider Epinephrine 0.3mg IM

Hereditary

- Congenital or acquired loss of C1 esterase inhibitor
- C1 inhibitor (C1INH), Ecallantide or Icatibant are all possible therapies

ACE-I induced

- ACEI adverse reaction from excessive bradykinin
- Administer FFP 2-4 units (contains multiple enzymes which degrade bradykinin) in severe cases or consider Icatibant for severe cases

Idiopathic

- Supportive care with consideration to all of the above therapies

CAT AND DOG BITES

- Coverage for Pasteurella, Strep, and Staph
- Amoxicillin-Clavulanate 875mg PO BID x 5-7 days or
- Doxycycline 100mg PO daily x 14 days if penicillin allergic or
- Clindamycin 450mg (5mg/kg) PO q8hrs daily x7 days and
    - Ciprofloxacin 500mg PO q12hrs x 7 days or
    - TMP/SMX 2DS tabs (5mg/kg) PO q12hrs

HUMAN BITES

- Coverage targets S. aureus, Strep Viridans, Bacteroides, Coagulase-neg Staph, Eikenella, Fusobacterium, Cornebacterium, Peptostreptococcus
    - Amoxicillin-Clavulanate 875mg PO BID x 5-7days or
    - Clindamycin 450mg (5mg/kg) PO q8hrs daily x7 days and
        - Ciprofloxacin 500mg PO q12hrs x 7 days or
        - TMP/SMX 2DS tabs (5mg/kg) PO q12hrs

ANTHRAX

Postexposure Prophylaxis

- Patient should be vaccinated at day #0, #14, #28
- Ciprofloxacin 500mg PO q12hrs daily x 60 days or
- Doxycycline 100mg PO q12hrs x 60 days

Cutaneous or inhalational disease

- Ciprofloxacin 400mg IV q12hrs x 60 days (1st line) or
- Doxycycline 100mg IV q12hrs x 60days (only if allergic to ciprofloxacin)

Pediatric Post-exposure Prophylaxis

- Ciprofloxacin 15mg/kg PO q12hrs x 60 days
- Doxycycline 2.2mg/kg PO q12hrs x 60 days

Pediatric Inhalational or Cutaneous

- Ciprofloxacin 15mg/kg IV q12hrs (1st line) or
- Doxycycline 2.2mg/kg IV q12hrs (only if allergic to cipro) and

- Clindamycin 7.5mg/kg q6hrs daily

Neurology

BELL'S PALSY

- Dysfunction of peripheral cranial nerve VII of unknown causing unilateral facial paralysis involving the forehead and lower face.
- Also associated with taste abnormalities: hyperacusis, decreased tearing, and subjective facial numbness.
- **Start steroids within 72hrs of symptom onset**
  - Prednisone 60-80mg qday x1wk
- **Antivirals offer little additional benefit when combined with steroids but also offer little harm**
  - Valacyclovir 1000mg TID x1 week or
  - Acyclovir 400mg 5x per day x1 week
- **Eye Protection and artificial tears can prevent unintended corneal abrasions in addition to ophthalmic ointment at night**

MIGRAINE HEADACHE

Headache attacks lasting 4–72 hr

- Unilateral location
- Pulsating quality
- Moderate or severe pain intensity
- Aggravation by or causing avoidance of routine physical activity
- Headaches associated with nausea/vomiting and/or
- Photophobia or phonophobia

Migraine treatment options

- Prochlorperazine (compazine) 10mg IV (first line)
- Metoclopramide (reglan) 10mg IV (second line)
- Ketorolac 10-15 mg IV (adjunctive therapy
- Dexamethasone 10mg IV can prevent recurrent migraines but does not provide acute pain relief

GUILLAIN-BARRE SYNDROME (GBS)

- **Ascending acute polyneuropathy (often immune-mediated) that presents with motor deficits in addition to sensory deficits.**
- Can be associated with acute infections from campylobacter jejuni, cytomegalovirus, Epstein-Barr virus, and Mycoplasma pneumoniae

GBS types

- **Acute inflammatory demyelinating polyneuropathy** - most common type with progressive symmetric muscle weakness
- **Acute motor axonal neuropathy** - often associated with campylobacter infections with only motor involvement
- **Acute motor and sensory axonal neuropathy** - both motor and sensory involvement
- **Miller-Fisher Syndrome** - descending paralysis with ophthalmoplegia with ataxia and areflexia

Lumbar puncture

- May show albumin-cytological dissociation of CSF (high protein (>45) and low WBC count (<10)
- Treat with IVIG and/or Plasmapheresis

Indication for emergent intubation include

- Vital capacity <15mL/kg
- Negative Inspiratory Force < 30 cm H2O
- PaO2 <70 mm Hg on room air
- Bulbar dysfunction (difficulty with breathing, swallowing, or speech)

MENINGITIS

- Organisms include pneumococcus, meningococcus, group B streptococcus, H. flu, listeria, or viral causes
- CSF cultures become sterile in 2 hrs after parenteral antibiotics in meningococcal meningitis and 6 hrs in pneumococcal meningitis
- Give dexamethasone 15 min prior to or with first dose of antibiotics (10mg IV q6hr x4d)
- Acyclovir - consider for suspected viral meningitis - 10mg/kg IV q8hr (

>1 month - Adults

- Ceftriaxone 2gm (50mg/kg) IV BID daily and

- Vancomycin 15-20 mg/kg IV BID daily

Neonates (up to 1 month of age)

- Ampicillin 50mg/kg IV q6hrs PLUS
- Cefotaxime 50mg/kg IV q6hrs OR Gentamicin 2.5mg/kg IV q8hrs

Cryptococcosis Meningitis

- Amphotericin B 1mg/kg IV once daily AND Flucytosine 25mg/kg PO q6hrs daily

LP RESULTS BY DISEASE

Measure	Normal	Bacterial	Aseptic (Viral)	Fungal	Tuberculosis	Subarachnoid hemorrhage	Neoplastic
Appearance	Clear	Clear, cloudy, or purulent	Clear	Clear or opaque	Clear or opaque	Xanthochromia, bloody, or clear	Clear or opaque
Opening Pressure (cm H2O)	10-20	>25	Normal or elevated	>25	>25	>25	Normal or elevated
WBC Count (cells/μL)	0-5	>100	5-1000	<500	50-500	0-5 (see correction section)	<500
% PMNs		>80-90%	1-50%^^	1-50%	Early PMN then lymph		1-50%
Glucose	>60% of serum glucose	Low	Normal	Low	Low	Normal	Normal
Protein^^^ (mg/dL)	< 45	Elevated	Elevated	Elevated	Elevated	Elevated	>200
Gram Stain	Neg	Pos	Neg	India ink	Tb stain	Blood	

MULTIPLE SCLEROSIS

- **Relapsing/remitting (most common) -** Relapse (days-months) followed by remission
- **Secondary progressive -** Relapses and partial recoveries occur, but disability does not fade away between cycles
- **Primary progressive -** Symptoms progress slowly and steadily without remission
- **Progressive relapsing -** Similar to primary progressive but with superimposed flares

- **Optic neuritis** - Initial sign in 30% of patients vision loss (usually unilateral) often preceded by retrobulbar pain
- **Internuclear ophthalmoplegia** - Abnormal eye adduction bilaterally and horizontal nystagmus
- **CSF** - demonstrates elevated protein and gamma-globulin (increased oligoclonal bands)
- **MRI** - multiple lesions in supratentorial white matter, paraventricular area, spinal cord
- **Initial treatment involves high-dose steroids (1gm solumedrol Q!2hrs)**

NORMAL PRESSURE HYDROCEPHALUS

- CSF buildup in the ventricles leading to increased intracranial pressure with edema of the periventricular white matter and corona radiata
- Gait disturbance is most common and earliest finding
- Diagnostic and therapeutic large volume CSF removal confirms the disease

STATUS EPILEPTICUS

- Patient seizing for 5-10min despite initial treatments

First line therapy

- Midazolam IM/IN 10 mg (> 40 kg) or 0.2 mg/kg
- Lorazepam IV 2 mg or 0.1 mg/kg
- Diazepam IV 0.15-0.2 mg/kg (up to 10 mg) or PR 0.2-0.5 mg/kg (up to 20 mg)

Second Line Therapy

- Fosphenytoin IV 20-30 mg/kg at 150 mg/min
- Levetiracetam IV 60 mg/kg, max 4500 mg/dose (preferred in pregnancy)

SUBARACHNOID HEMORRHAGE (SAH)

- Bleeding into the subarachnoid space, between the arachnoid membrane and the pia mater.
- Can occur from trauma or spontaneously, from a ruptured aneurysm
  - Requires seizure prophylaxis and neurosurgery consult

- **Within 6 hours of severe headache a CT non-con of the brain van rule out SAH with 99-100% sensitivity**
- LP results show elevated RBC count that does not decrease meaningfully from tube one to four
- Xanthochromia - occurs many hours after bleeding but may help differentiate SAH from a traumatic LP
- **A CT followed by CTA is an acceptable alternative to CT and LP to determine if the patient has aneurysms at risk of of rupture**

TRANSVERSE MYELITIS

- Inflammatory disorder that involves a complete transverse section of the spinal cord
- Can present with vague spinal neurologic complaint or classic bilateral motor, sensory, and autonomic disturbances
- MRI is required for diagnosis and rule out of compressive masses

TRIGEMINAL NEURALGIA

- Paroxysms of severe unilateral pain in trigeminal nerve distribution lasting seconds to minutes
- Carbamazepine (first line)
  - Decreases the response of neurons to peripheral stimulation
  - Initial dose at 100mg one to two times per da increase by 100-200mg every 3 days
- Initial evaluation can involve a CT face to assess for compressive facial lesions

SPINAL CORD SYNDROMES

- Complete spinal cord transection syndrome
- Anterior cord syndrome
- Central cord syndrome
- Brown-Sequard syndrome
- **Epidural compression syndromes**
  - Syringomyelia
  - Spinal cord compression (non-traumatic)
  - Cauda equina syndrome

- Conus medullaris syndrome
- Epidural abscess (spinal)
- Epidural hematoma (spinal)

BROWN-SEQUARD SYNDROME

- Transverse hemisection of spinal cord
- Decussation of corticospinal tract at the medulla and complete lack of decussation of fibers of the posterior columns result in:
  - **Ipsilateral spastic paresis**
  - **Ipsilateral loss of proprioception and vibration**
  - **Contralateral loss of pain, temperature (sensory dissociation)**
- Requires emergent neurosurgery consult

SPINAL EPIDURAL ABSCESS

- Usually spans up to 3-5 vertebral spaces as an abscess confined to epidural adipose tissue in spine.
- MRI with and without contrast should be performed regardless of the suspected spinal level

Causative organisms include

- **S. aureus (and MRSA)**
- **S. epidermidis (post surgery)**
- **E. coli**
- **P. aeruginosa (IVDA)**

Most common physical exam findings

- **Fever**
- **Spinal tenderness**
- **Sensory or motor deficit**
- **Reflex abnormality or rectal tone decrease**

Antibiotic therapy (plus neuro surgical consult)

- **Vancomycin 15-20mg/kg BID and metronidazole 500g (7.5mg/kg) q6 hrs and (Cefotaxime or Ceftriaxone or Ceftazidime)**

CAUDA EQUINA SYNDROME

- The cauda equina ("horse's tail") begins at L2 (below conus medullaris) and extends down to the sacral nerves.
- **Often presents with severe asymmetric sudden pain in radicular distribution in addition to:**
  - Saddle anesthesia
  - Decreased motor strength
  - Urinary retention (with or without incontinence)
  - Unilateral or bilateral sensory deficits
- **Ideal workup should include an MRI non-contrast of the lumbar/ sacral spine**

CONUS MEDULLARIS SYNDROME

- Lesions at vertebral level L2 with bilateral symptoms (directly above the cauda equina)
- will present will all of the symptoms of cauda equina and more likely to have bilateral symptoms

ACUTE ISCHEMIC STROKE

- **Non-con CT head can be normal up to six hours post-stroke**

Internal Capsule and Lacunar Infarcts

- May present with either lacunar pure motor or pure sensory (of face and body)

Anterior Circulation

- Blood supply via internal carotid system
- Includes ACA and MCA
- **Anterior Cerebral Artery (ACA) occlusion**
  - Contralateral sensory and motor symptoms in the lower extremity (sparing hands/face)
- **Middle Cerebral Artery (MCA) occlusion**
  - Hemiparesis, facial plegia, sensory loss contralateral to affected cortex

- Motor deficits found more commonly in face and upper extremity than lower extremity

Posterior circulation

- Blood supply via the vertebral artery
- Branches include, AICA, Basilar artery, PCA and PICA
- 5 Ds: Dizziness (Vertigo), Dysarthria, Dystaxia, Diplopia, Dysphagia
- Crossed neuro deficits (i.e., ipsilateral CN deficits with contralateral motor weakness)
- **Superior Cerebellar Artery (SCA)**
  - Nonspecific symptoms - N/V, dizziness, ataxia, nystagmus
- **Posterior Cerebral Artery (PCA)**
  - Visual field defects (contralateral homonymous hemianopsia, unilateral blindness)
  - Rarely with motor involvement
  - Medial midbrain syndrome - ipsilateral CN III with contralateral paralysis of face, arm, leg
  - Lateral midbrain syndrome - Ipsilateral CN III with contralateral hemiataxia, tremor, hyperkinesis
- **Basilar artery occlusion**
  - Quadriplegia, coma, locked-in syndrome
- **Anterior Inferior Cerebellar Artery (AICA) occlusion**
  - Ipsilateral facial paralysis, loss of corneal reflex (CN VII), ipsilateral loss of pain/temp (CN V), and ipsilateral limb and gait ataxia
  - Ipsilateral Horner syndrome
- **Posterior Inferior Cerebellar Artery (PICA)**
  - Ipsilateral cerebellar signs, ipsilateral loss of pain/temp of face, ipsilateral Horner's syndrome, ipsilateral dysphagia and hoarseness, dysarthria, vertigo/nystagmus

Thrombolysis for acute CVA

- Goal SBP to < 185 mmHg
- tPA if no bleeding or other contraindications AND if less than 3 hours from symptom onset

tPA contraindications

- Stroke or head trauma in previous 3 months
- History of intracranial hemorrhage
- Major surgery in the previous 14 days
- GI or urinary bleeding in previous 21 days
- Rapid resolution of stroke symptoms
- Persistent SBP >185 or DBP >110 despite treatment
- Anticoagulation
- Hypoglycemia
- ICH visible on head CT
- Intracranial mass, AVM, or aneurysm

ACUTE THROMBECTOMY OF LARGE VESSEL OCCLUSION

- **"Cortical strokes" of ICA, MCA, and some ACA occlusions are most likely to benefit from thrombectomy**
- CT perfusion study is the key factor in determining brain tissue salvageability from symptom onset to thrombectomy of 6-24 hours

ACUTE HEMORRHAGIC STROKE

- Rapid SBP lowering <140mmHg has been advocated but more recent work has found no difference between SBP <140 mmHg and <180 mmHg
- If lowering blood pressure utilize the following options
    - **Nicardipine - 5mg/hr initial increased q5min by 2.5mg until target blood pressure then titrate down to infusion of 3mg/hr or**
    - **Labetolol - 20mg initial and then 20mg q3-5 mins until target blood pressure hen start an infusion of 1-8mg/min.**
- Workup is focused on identifying the underlying etiology causing the ICH and maintaining stability:
    - Avoid Hypotension
    - Prevent Seizures
    - Reverse coagulopathy
    - Elevated head of bed 30 degrees

TRANSIENT ISCHEMIC ATTACK (CVA)

New Definition

- A brief episode of neurologic dysfunction caused by focal brain or retinal ischemia, with clinical symptoms typically lasting less than one hour, and without evidence of acute infarction on imaging

Classic Definition

- A sudden, focal neurologic deficit that lasts for less than 24 hours, is presumed to be of vascular origin, and is confined to an area of the brain or eye perfused by a specific artery.
- Many CVAs are preceded by TIAs
- **ACEP Guidelines - Level B: In adult patients with suspected TIA, do not rely on current existing risk stratification instruments (eg, age, blood pressure, clinical features, duration of TIA and presence of diabetes, ABCD2 score) to identify TIA patients who can be safely discharged from the ED.**
- Evaluate for CHF and carotid stenosis.

CEREBRAL VENOUS SINUS THROMBOSIS

- Occlusion of venous sinus (most commonly superior sagittal and lateral sinuses) by thrombus
- **Although presentation can be highly variable, neurodefecits can be correlated with the location of the occlusion**
    - **Superior sagital sinus** - motor deficits, seizures
    - **Left transverse sinus** - aphasia
    - **Cavernous sinus** - ocular pain, protosis, oculomotor palsies
    - **Deep venous sinus** - thalamic and basal ganglia related symptoms such as altered mental status
- Risk factors include: cancer, pregnancy, infections (otitis media, sinusitis, cellulitis, dental infections), hypercoagulable states, trauma
- Diagnosis can often be accomplished with a CTV if MRI/MRV is unavailable.

NEUROCYSTICERCOSIS

Albendazole

- First line therapy:15mg/kg/day divided in 2 doses

Praziquantel

- Second line therapy: 50-100mg/kg/day divided in 3 doses

Rocky Mountain Spotted Fever

- Doxycycline 100 mg BID for 5-7 days
- Indicated also in children at 2.2mg/kg BID
- Chloramphenicol (CAM) 50-100 mg/kg/day div Q6hr (Max dose = 4g/day)
- Preferred agent in pregnancy. May cause aplastic anemia and Grey baby syndrome, more common in near term or 3rd trimester
- Consideration should be made for doxycycline over CAM in the 3rd trimester

BRAIN ABSCESS

Otogenic source

- Cefotaxime 2gm IV q6hr + metronidazole 500mg IV q6hr

Sinogenic or odontogenic source

- Cefotaxime 2gm IV q6hr + metronidazole 500mg IV q6hr

Penetrating trauma or neurosurgical procedures

- Vancomycin 15mg/kg IV q12hr + ceftazidime 2gm IV q8hr

Hematogenous source

- Cefotaxime 2gm IV q6hr + metronidazole 500mg IV q6hr

No obvious source

- Cefotaxime 2gm IV q6hr + metronidazole 500mg IV q6hr

ENCEPHALITIS

- Often it is unclear which type of encephalitis is present and starting Acyclovir empirically is appropriate. In addition to the pathogens below, possible causes can include West Nile Virus, EBV, HIV, toxoplasmosis, or rabies.

HSV encephalitis

- Acyclovir 10mg/kg (10-15mg/kg for pediatrics) every 8hrs

HZV encephalitis

- Acyclovir 10mg/kg every 8hr

CMV encephalitis

- Ganciclovir 5mg/kg IV every 12hr or
- Foscarnet 90mg/kg IV every 12 hrs

Tick Associated (Borrelia, Ehrlichia or Rickettsia)

- Doxycycline 200 mg IV once followed by 100 mg IV twice daily

EPIDURAL ABSCESS

- Target Staph, Strep, and Gram-negative bacilli
- Vancomycin 15-20mg/kg BID and metronidazole 500g (7.5mg/kg) q6 hrs and (Cefotaxime or Ceftriaxone or Ceftazidime)
- Ceftazidime is preferred if pseudomonas is considered likely
- Can substitute Nafcillin or Oxacillin for Vancomycin if not MRSA
- Treat for 6-8 weeks

MENINGITIS

Neonates (up to 1 month of age)

- Ampicillin 50mg/kg IV q6hrs and
- Cefotaxime 50mg/kg IV q6hrs or Gentamicin 2.5mg/kg IV q8hrs

Greater than 1 month old

- Ceftriaxone 2gm (50mg/kg) IV BID daily and
- Vancomycin 15-20 mg/kg IV BID daily
- Vancomycin is for resistant Pneumococcus
- For the elderly or immunocompromised adults, add Ampicillin 2gm IV q4h (for listeria coverage)

Obstetrics and Gynecology

MASTITIS

- No need to routinely interrupt breastfeeding with puerperal mastitis.
- For mild symptoms <24 hours, supportive care may be sufficient
- Effective milk removal (frequent breast feeding - use pumping to augment milk removal)
- Analgesia (NSAIDs)

Antibiotics

- Treatment directed at S. aureus and Strep and E. coli
- Uncomplicated mastitis → 10 days of antibiotics (regardless of MRSA suspicion)
- Dicloxacillin 500mg PO q6hrs, considered first line if breastfeeding given safety for infant or
- Cephalexin 500mg PO q6hrs or
- Add TMP/SMX 2DS tabs PO q12hrs if suspect MRSA
- Clindamycin 450mg PO q8hrs (also provides MRSA coverage) or
- Amoxicillin/Clavulanate 875mg PO q12hrs or
- Azithromycin 500mg PO x1 on day 1, then 250mg PO daily for days 2-5

BARTHOLIN'S CYST

- Occurs when Bartholin's gland within the labia, becomes blocked
- They are usually between 1 and 4 cm, and are located just medial to the labia minora

ENDOMETRITIS

<48hrs Post Partum

- Treatment is targeted against polymicrobial infections, most often 2-3 organisms of normal vaginal flora
- Clindamycin 900mg q8hrs and Gentamicin 1.5mg/kg IV q8hrs or
- Doxycycline 100mg IV PO q12hrs daily and

- Ampicillin/Sulbactam 3g IV q6hrs
- Cefoxitin 2g IV q6hrs daily

>48hrs Post Partum

- Doxycycline 100mg IV or PO q12hrs and Metronidazole 500mg IV or PO q8hrs daily

PID

- If possible, treat all partners who had sex with patient during previous 60 days prior to symptom onset

Outpatient Options

- Ceftriaxone 250mg IM (or IV) x1 and doxycycline 100mg PO BID x14d and/or metronidazole 500mg PO BID x14d
- Metronidazole based upon assessment of risk for anaerobes; consider in:
- Pelvic abscess
- Proven or suspected infection w/ Trichomonas or Bacterial Vaginosis
- History of gynecological instrumentation in the preceding 2-3wks
- Cefoxitin 2 g IM in a single dose and Probenecid, 1 g PO administered concurrently in a single dose and Doxycycline 100 mg PO BID x 14 days and/or flagyl based on above criteria

Alternative Outpatient Options

- Ceftriaxone 250mg IM x1 and 1 g of azithromycin per week, x 2 weeks and/or flagyl based on above criteria
- A single randomized controlled trial shows that azithromycin is superior to doxycycline even when compliance in taking doxycycline is excellent (98.2% vs 87.5%)

Inpatient

- Cefoxitin 2gm IV q6hr or cefotetan 2gm IV q12hr) and doxycycline PO or IV 100 mg q12hr or
- Clindamycin 900mg IV q8h and gentamicin 2mg/kg QD or
- Ampicillin-sulbactam 3gm IV q6hr and doxycycline 100mg IV/PO q12hr

CANDIDA VAGINITIS

Intravaginal Therapy

- Clotrimazole 1 % cream applied vaginally for 7 days or
- Clotrimazole 2% applied vaginally for 3 days or

Oral Therapy

- Fluconazole 150mg PO once
- A second dose at 72hrs can be given if patient is still symptomatic

Pregnant Patients

- Intravaginal Clotrimazole or Miconazole are the only recommended treatments
- Duration is 7 days
- PO fluconazole associated with congenital malformations and spontaneous abortions

CERVICITIS

- Treatment to cover both gonorrhea and chlamydia
  - Ceftriaxone 250mg IM once and
  - Azithromycin 1g PO once or
  - Doxycycline 100mg PO BID x 14 days

Cephalosporin Allergy

- Azithromycin 2g PO once and
- Gentamicin 240mg IM once

BACTERIAL VAGINOSIS OR TRICHOMONAS

- Metronidazole 2g PO
- If pregnant, avoid breast feeding until 24-hrs after dose

ECTOPIC PREGNANCY

- Leading cause of maternal death in first trimester and overall third leading cause of maternal death

- Occur in 2% of all pregnancies and as high as 6-16% in those presenting to the ED
- Pregnancy in patient with prior tubal ligation or IUD in place is ectopic until proven otherwise (25-50% are ectopic)

Risk Factor	Odds Ratio
Previous tubal surgery	21
Previous ectopic pregnancy	8.3
Diethylstilbestrol exposure	5.6
Previous PID	2.4 to 3.7
Assisted Fertility	2 to 2.5
Smoker	2.3
Previous intrauterine device use	1.6

Algorithm for Ectopic evaluation

- **Step one**
  - Assess for Shock
  - Beware that paradoxical bradycardia can be present with significant hemoperitoneum
  - If patient is a high risk for ectopic based on above estimation then immediately contact OBGYN
- **Step Two**
  - Perform a Pelvic US
  - Consider Transabdominal Ultrasound for B-HCG: >6000 mIU/ml (but if negative or indeterminate must do Pelvic ultrasound regardless of B-HCG)
  - If there is an IUP and there was no assisted reproductive fertility used then ectopic ruled out and heterotopic unlikely (less than 1:30,000)
  - If fertility assistance was used then still consider a heterotopic (1% risk
- **Step Three**

- If HCG above Discriminatory Zone (>1,500-3,000 mIU/ml) and not visualized it should be an ectopic pregnancy until proven otherwise

- **Step Four**
  - Arrange close follow-up for patients with no visualized IUP and B-HCG((<1,500-3,000 mIU/ml), with minimal to no pain and hemodynamically stable.
  - Patients should have a 48hr repeat B-HCG level checked to determine if appropriate doubling is occurring.

Treatment and Management

- RhoGAM for all Rh-negative women and OB/GYN consult for all ectopic00.Medical management with methotrexate (ACOG)
- **Medical management with methotrexate (ACOG)**
  - Methotrexate 50mg/m2 IM day 1
  - If hCG decreases by <15% between days 4 and 7, another 50mg IM methotrexate on day 7
- **Absolute contraindications**
  - Breast-feeding
  - Laboratory evidence of immunodeficiency
  - Preexisting blood dyscrasia (bone marrow hypoplasia, leukopenia, thrombocytopenia, or clinically significant anemia)
  - Known sensitivity to methotrexate
  - Active pulmonary disease
  - Peptic ulcer disease
  - Hepatic, renal, or hematologic dysfunction
  - Alcoholism
  - Alcoholic or other chronic liver disease
  - Coexistant viable IUP
  - Does not have timely access to medical institution, or unwilling/unable to comply with post-MTX monitoring
- **Surgical treatment**
  - Urgent laparotomy if patient is unstable
  - Otherwise, laparoscopic salpingectomy or salpingostomy can be done

POSTPARTUM ENDOMETRITIS

- Inflammation of the endometrial lining of the uterus.
- Endometritis can be divided into pregnancy-related endometritis and endometritis unrelated to pregnancy. When the condition is unrelated to pregnancy, it is referred to as pelvic inflammatory disease (PID)

<48hrs Post Partum

Treatment is targeted against polymicrobial infections
- Clindamycin 900mg q8hrs PLUS Gentamicin 1.5mg/kg IV q8hrs OR
- Doxycycline 100mg IV PO q12hrs daily PLUS
    - Ampicillin/Sulbactam 3g IV q6hrs
    - Cefoxitin 2g IV q6hrs daily

>48hrs Post Partum

- Doxycycline 100mg IV or PO q12hrs + Metronidazole 500mg IV or PO q8hrs daily

NON-PREGNANT VAGINAL BLEEDING

Systemic Causes

- Cirrhosis
- Coagulopathy (Von Willebrand, ITP)
- Group A strep vaginitis (prepubertal girls)
- Hormone replacement therapy
- Hypothyroidism
- Secondary anovulation

Reproductive Tract Causes

- Dysfunctional uterine bleeding
- Endometriosis
- Fibroids
- Foreign Body
- Infection (vaginitis, PID)

- IUD
- Neoplasia
- Vaginal Trauma

VAGINAL BLEEDING IN PREGNANCY (<20 WEEKS) DIFFERENTIAL

- Ectopic pregnancy
- First Trimester Abortion
  - Complete Abortion
  - Incomplete Abortion
  - Inevitable Abortion
  - Missed Abortion
  - Septic abortion
  - Threatened Abortion
- Gestational trophoblastic disease
- Heterotopic pregnancy
- Implantation bleeding
- Molar pregnancy

VAGINAL BLEEDING IN PREGNANCY (>20WEEKS) DIFFERENTIAL

- Placental abruption
- Placenta previa
- Vasa previa
- Uterine rupture
- Preterm labor
- Vaginal trauma
- Placenta accreta
- Intrauterine fetal demise

SPONTANEOUS ABORTION

- RhoGam if Rh Negative

- IVF and/or PRBCs if severe bleeding
- Misoprostol only for < 12 weeks gestation, high success rate for the following[1]
- Incomplete AB: 600 mcg PO single dose
- Missed AB: 800 mcg vaginally single dose
- Supportive care with anti-emetic and NSAIDs for misoprostol side effects
- D&C and OB/gyn consult may be necessary if medical management fails or continuous products/vaginal bleeding > 7-14 days

	Characteristics	OS	Fetal Tissue Passage	Misc
Threatened	Abdominal pain or bleeding; < 20 weeks gestation	Closed	No	If < 11 weeks (with fetal cardiac activity) 90% progress to term. If between 11 and 20 weeks 50% progress to term
Inevitable	Abdominal pain or bleeding; < 20 weeks gestation	Open	No	
Incomplete	Abdominal pain or bleeding; < 20 weeks gestation	Open	Yes, some	
Complete	Abdominal pain or bleeding; < 20 weeks gestation	Closed	Yes, complete expulsion of products	Distinguish from ectopic based on decreasing hCG and/or decreased bleeding
Missed	Fetal death at <20 weeks without passage of any fetal tissue for 4 weeks after fetal death	Closed	No	
Septic	Infection of the uterus during a miscarriage. Most commonly caused by retained products of conception	Open	No, or may be incomplete	Uterine tenderness and purulent discharge from the OS may be present

OVARIAN TORSION

- Ovarian torsion is the rotation of the ovary and portion of the fallopian tube on the supplying vascular pedicle
- Referred to as adnexal torsion and tubo-ovarian torsion
- Occurs in females of all ages
- Most common in reproductive age adults
- In children, it is most common in 9-14 years of age
- **Risk factors:**
  - Ovarian mass
  - Fertility treatments
  - Ovarian cysts (usually > 4 cm) and neoplasms account for 94% of cases in adults
- Torsion more common on the right, as the sigmoid colon tends to stabilize the left
- In children, hypermobility of the ovary many be the primary cause of torsion
- Dual blood supply from ovarian and uterine arteries

Doppler ultrasound torsion findings:
  - Diminished or absent blood flow in the ovarian vessels
  - 2/3 of patients with ovarian torsion have had normal blood flow
  - Venous and lymphatic obstruction occurs before arterial disruption, especially early in disease process
  - Abnormal blood flow, whether venous or arterial, is ~85% sensitive, ~37% specific when not combined with below findings
  - Ovarian mass > 3 cm may be clue
  - Enlarged ovarian volume
- **CT Abd/Pelvis**
  - CT has a low sensitivity for torsion
    - Examine for asymmetric ovarian enlargement, which warrants a pelvic US if concerning symptoms exist
  - CT may be used to rule out other possible causes of lower abdominal pain; also exclude presence of pelvic mass

PLACENTAL ABRUPTION

- Premature separation of placenta from uterus
- Usually occurs spontaneously but also associated with trauma (even minor trauma)
- Usually occurs at >15 weeks gestation
- Must be considered in patients who presenting with painful vaginal bleeding near term
- Abruption may be complete, partial, or concealed
  - Amount of external bleeding may not correlate with severity
- **Risk Factors**
  - Hypertension
  - Trauma
  - Smoking
  - Advanced maternal age
  - Multiparity
  - Preeclampsia
  - Prior placental abruption
  - Thrombophilia
  - Cocaine abuse
  - History of C-section or other uterine symptoms
- Requires emergent OBGYN consult and blood transfusion if hypotensive

PREECLAMPSIA

- Can occur after 20wks gestation and up to 4wk post-partum
- **Diagnosis is either based on blood pressure AND proteinuria or the presence of Severe Symptoms**
  - Systolic ≥140 mmHg or diastolic ≥90 mmHg on 2 occasions at least 4 hours apart, after 20 weeks gestation with previously normal BPs
  - Systolic ≥160 mmHg or diastolic ≥110 mmHg acutely requiring emergent blood pressure decreases
  - Proteinuria ≥300mg in a 24-hour urine collection
  - Spot protein(mg/dL)/creatinine(mg/dL) ratio ≥0.3
  - **Severe Symptoms:**

- Platelets <100,000/mL
- Elevated LFTS
- New renal insufficiency (creatinine >1.1mg/dL or doubling of creatinine concentration in absence of renal disease)
- Pulmonary edema
- New onset visual complaints
- ED diagnosis and recognition requires urgent obgyn consult or referral

ECLAMPSIA

- Onset of seizures in a pregnant woman with pre-eclampsia
- Definitive therapy is delivery
- **Immediately administer magnesium: Load 6 g IV over 15 min followed by 2-3 gm/hr**
    - **If no IV access then use 10 gm IM (5 g in each buttock)**
- Labetalol or Hydralazine should target a blood pressure of SBP<130mmHg
- Benzodiazepines can treat refractory seizures

POSTPARTUM EMERGENCIES

- **Amniotic fluid embolus**
    - Cardiac or respiratory arrest occuring during labor or within 30 minutes of delivery
- **Chorioamnionitis**
    - Septic appearing pregnant women after first trimester
- **Eclampsia**
- **HELLP syndrome**
    - Hemolysis, Elevated LFTs, Low Platelets
- **Mastitis**
- **Peripartum cardiomyopathy**
- **Postpartum endometritis**
- **Postpartum hemorrhage**
- **Preeclampsia**
- **Retained products of conception**

- Premature separation of placenta from uterus
- Usually occurs spontaneously but also associated with trauma (even minor trauma)
- Usually occurs at >15 weeks gestation
- Must be considered in patients who presenting with painful vaginal bleeding near term
- Abruption may be complete, partial, or concealed
  - Amount of external bleeding may not correlate with severity
- **Risk Factors**
  - Hypertension
  - Trauma
  - Smoking
  - Advanced maternal age
  - Multiparity
  - Preeclampsia
  - Prior placental abruption
  - Thrombophilia
  - Cocaine abuse
  - History of C-section or other uterine symptoms
- Requires emergent OBGYN consult and blood transfusion if hypotensive

PREECLAMPSIA

- Can occur after 20wks gestation and up to 4wk post-partum
- **Diagnosis is either based on blood pressure AND proteinuria or the presence of Severe Symptoms**
  - Systolic ≥140 mmHg or diastolic ≥90 mmHg on 2 occasions at least 4 hours apart, after 20 weeks gestation with previously normal BPs
  - Systolic ≥160 mmHg or diastolic ≥110 mmHg acutely requiring emergent blood pressure decreases
  - Proteinuria ≥300mg in a 24-hour urine collection
  - Spot protein(mg/dL)/creatinine(mg/dL) ratio ≥0.3
  - **Severe Symptoms:**

- Platelets <100,000/mL
- Elevated LFTS
- New renal insufficiency (creatinine >1.1mg/dL or doubling of creatinine concentration in absence of renal disease)
- Pulmonary edema
- New onset visual complaints
- ED diagnosis and recognition requires urgent obgyn consult or referral

ECLAMPSIA

- Onset of seizures in a pregnant woman with pre-eclampsia
- Definitive therapy is delivery
- **Immediately administer magnesium: Load 6 g IV over 15 min followed by 2-3 gm/hr**
  - **If no IV access then use 10 gm IM (5 g in each buttock)**
- Labetalol or Hydralazine should target a blood pressure of SBP<130mmHg
- Benzodiazepines can treat refractory seizures

POSTPARTUM EMERGENCIES

- **Amniotic fluid embolus**
  - Cardiac or respiratory arrest occuring during labor or within 30 minutes of delivery
- **Chorioamnionitis**
  - Septic appearing pregnant women after first trimester
- **Eclampsia**
- **HELLP syndrome**
  - Hemolysis, Elevated LFTs, Low Platelets
- **Mastitis**
- **Peripartum cardiomyopathy**
- **Postpartum endometritis**
- **Postpartum hemorrhage**
- **Preeclampsia**
- **Retained products of conception**

• Uterine rupture

HELLP SYNDROME

Hemolysis

• Microangiopathic hemolytic anemia (Schistocytes on microscopy)

Elevated LFTs

• AST ALT elevation and often elevated, bilirubin

Low Platelets

• Platelet count < 150 × 109 per L

COMMON POSTPARTUM EMERGENCIES

• Amniotic fluid embolus
• Chorioamnionitis
• Eclampsia
• HELLP syndrome
• Mastitis
• Peripartum cardiomyopathy
• Postpartum endometritis
• Postpartum headache
• Postpartum hemorrhage
• Preeclampsia
• Retained products of conception
• Uterine rupture

POSTPARTUM HEMORRHAGE

• Leading cause of maternal death worldwide and caused by:
    • **Uterine atony (responsible for 80% of cases)**
    • **Retained placental tissue**
    • **Lower genital tract lacerations**
    • **Uterine rupture**

- **Uterine inversion**
- **Underlying coagulation abnormalities**
- Early tranexamic acid (TXA) reduces death due to bleeding
- Give as soon as possible relative to bleeding onset
- 1 g IV of TXA over 10 min, with 2nd dose 30 min later if continual bleed OR bleed restarts within 24 hrs after 1st dose

Uterine atony (boggy uterus) treatment options

- **Bimanual Massage**
- **Oxytocin (Pitocin)** - 1st line and most important drug - Oxytocin 80 units in 500 cc NS bag, run it wide open or
- **Misoprostol (Cytotec) -** 600mcg SL or 1000 mcg rectally
- **Methylergonovine (Methergine)** - 0.2mg IM q2-4 hrs (relative contraindication in patients with hypertension or Preeclampsia - may consider in severely unstable BP)
- **Carboprost (Hemabate)** - 250mcg IM q15 min (avoid in patients with asthma)
- **Bakri balloon** - placement, fill with warm 500ml NS (or large/multiple Foleys or pack) - use US to place to top of fundus and ensure no retained placenta

Traumatic causes

- **Genital tract tear**
    - Suture lacerations - figure of eight with 3-0 or 2-0 absorbable
    - Deep lacerations such as those by the cervix may require OR
    - Drain hematomas >3 cm
- **Uterine inversion**
    - Manually replace placenta OR do not remove placenta until uterus has been replaced:
    - Place hand inside the vagina and push the fundus cephalad along long axis of vagina
    - Prompt replacement important since cervix contracts over time creating a constriction ring
    - **Discontinue uterotonic meds (oxytocin)** if uterus not reduced, and consider uterine relaxant options:[6]:

- Nitroglycerine IV 50-250 mcg bolus over 1-2 min, then up to x3-4 additional doses q3-5 min to relax uterus
- Magnesium 4-6 g IV over 15 min
- Terbutaline 0.25mg IV or SQ
- **After uterine reversion and reduction:**
  - Fundal massage ± bimanual massage/compression
  - Then oxytocin infusion with 40 units in 1 L of NS at 200-1000 cc/hr

Genitourinary

URETHRITIS (MALE)

- Treatment to cover both gonorrhea and chlamydia:
  - **Ceftriaxone 250mg IM once, and**
  - **Azithromycin 1g PO once or**
  - **Doxycycline 100mg PO BID x 7 days**
- If cephalosporin Allergy then the regimen can be:
  - **Azithromycin 2g PO once, and**
  - **Gentamicin 240mg IM once**
- Consider coverage of trichomonas, among men who have sex with women
  - **Metronidazole 2 gm PO x 1, or**
  - **Tinidazole 2 gm PO x 1**

ACUTE CYSTITIS

- UTI therapy should rely on local antibiogram sensitivities as resistance patterns vary greatly

Women (Uncomplicated)

- Nitrofurantoin ER 100mg BID x 5d, or
- TMP/SMX DS (160/800mg) 1 tab BID x 3d, or
- Cephalexin 250mg QID x 5d, or
- Fosfomycin 3 g PO once
  - Fosfomycin may have lower cure success compared to nitrofurantoin for 5 days

Women (Complicated)

- Ciprofloxacin 500mg BID x10-14d, or
- Cefpodoxime 200 mg BID x10-14d

Men

- Ciprofloxacin 500mg BID x10-14d, or
- Cefpodoxime 200 mg BID x10-14d

PROSTATITIS

STD associated

- Doxycycline 100mg PO q12 hrs x14 days and
  - Ceftriaxone 250mg IM x1

No Associated STDs

- Therapy targeting E. coli and pseudomonas
  - Ciprofloxacin 500mg PO q12hrs x 28 days or
  - TMP/SMX 1 DS tablet PO q12hrs x 28 days
  - Consider extension to 6 wks of empiric therapy

PYELONEPHRITIS

- Treatment is targeted at E. coli, Enterococcus, Klebsiella, Proteus, S. saprophyticus

Outpatient Options

- Ciprofloxacin 500mg PO BID x7 days or
- Cefpodoxime 200mg PO BID x 10 days or
- Cefixime 400mg PO daily x 10 days or
- Levofloxacin 750mg PO QD x7 days

Inpatient Options

- Ciprofloxacin 400mg IV q12hr or
- Ceftriaxone 1gm IV QD or
- Cefotaxime 1-2gm IV q8hr or
- Gentamicin 3mg/kg/day divided q8hr and/or ampicillin 1–2 gm q4hr or
- Piperacillin/Tazobactam 3.375 gm IV q6hr or
- Cefepime 2gm IV q8hr or
- Imipenem 500mg IV q8hr

Pediatric Inpatient Options

- Ceftriaxone 75mg/kg IV QD or
- Cefotaxime 50mg/kg IV q8hrs or
- Ampicillin 25mg/kg IV q6hrs + Gentamicin 2.5mg/kg IV q8hrs

BALANOPOSTHITIS

Antifungal

- Clotrimazole 1% applied topically to glans q12hrs until resolution
- Nystatin cream 100,000 units/gm if infection is recurrent after clotrimazole therapy

Antibacterial

- Topical triple antibiotic ointment QID or mupirocin cream BID

EPIDIDYMITIS AND EPIDIDYMO-ORCHITIS

For acute epididymitis likely caused by STI

- Ceftriaxone 250 mg IM in a single dose and
- Doxycycline 100 mg orally twice a day for 10 days

If STD or enteric organisms (anal intercorse)

- Ceftriaxone 250 mg IM in a single dose and
- Levofloxacin 500 mg orally once a day for 10 days or
- Ofloxacin 300 mg orally twice a day for 10 days

Ophthalmology

PERIORBITAL SWELLING DIFFERENTIAL

Proptosis

- **Normal IOP**
    - Orbital cellulitis
    - Orbital pseudotumor
    - Orbital tumor
- **Increased IOP**
    - Retrobulbar abscess
    - Retrobulbar emphysema
    - Retrobulbar hemorrhage
    - Orbital tumor

No proptosis

- Periorbital cellulitis/erysipelas
- Dacryocystitis (lacrimal duct)
- Dacryocele/Dacryocystocele
- Dacryostenosis
- Dacryoadenitis (lacrimal gland)
- Allergic reaction
- Nephrotic Syndrome (pediatrics)

Lid Complications

- Blepharitis (crusts)
- Chalazion (meibomian gland)
- Stye (hordeolum) (eyelash follicle)

Other Causes

- Subperiosteal abscess
- Orbital abscess
- Cavernous sinus thrombosis
- Conjunctivitis

- Contact dermatitis
- Herpes zoster
- Herpes simplex
- Sarcoidosis
- Granulomatosis with polyangiitis

CORNEAL ABRASION

Non-contact lens wearer

- Erythromycin ointment qid x 3-5d or
- Ciprofloxacin 0.3% ophthalmic solution 2 drops q6 hours or
- Ofloxacin 0.3% solution 2 drops q6 hours or
- Sulfacetamide 10% ophthalmic ointment q6 hours

Contact lens wearer

- Antibiotics should cover pseudomonas and favor 3rd or 4th generation fluoroquinolones
    - Levofloxacin 0.5% solution 2 drops ever 2 hours for 2 days THEN q6hrs for 5 days or
    - Moxifloxacin 0.5% solution 2 drops every 2 hours for 2 days THEN q6hrs for 5 days or
    - Tobramycin 0.3% solution 2 drops q6hrs for 5 days or
    - Gentamicin 0.3% solution 2 drops six times for 5 days

ORBITAL CELLULITIS

- Vancomycin 15-20mg/kg IV BID and
    - Ampicillin/Sulbactam 3 g IV q6hr or
    - Ticarcillin/Clavulanate 3.1 g IV q4h or
    - Piperacillin-Tazobactam 4.5 g IV q6h or
    - Ceftriaxone 2 g IV q12hr or
    - Cefotaxime 2 g IV q4h

PERIORBITAL CELLULITIS

Outpatient

- Amoxicillin/Clavulanate 875mg BID x7-10 days or
- Cefpodoxime 200mg BID x7-10d or
- Cephalexin 450mg PO three times daily or
- Cefdinir 600mg PO once daily x7-10 days

Inpatient

- Vancomycin 15-20mg/kg IV BID and
    - Ampicillin/Sulbactam 3 g IV q6hr or
    - Piperacillin-Tazobactam 4.5 g IV q6h or
    - Ceftriaxone 2 g IV q12hr or
    - Cefotaxime 2 g IV q4h

BLEPHARITIS

- Inflammation of lid margin with ocular irritation, matted lashes
- **Distinguish anterior from posterior blepharitis using slit lamp**
    - Posterior - swelling and plugging of meibomian gland openings
    - Anterior - on external exam, material such as greasy flakes (seborrheic) or hard crust (staph) surrounds eyelashes
- **Treatment:**
    - Lid hygiene most important for both anterior and posterior blepharitis
    - Avoid eye-makeup
    - Warm compresses 15min 4x/day

KERATOCONJUNCTIVITIS

- Defined as concurrent inflammation of both the cornea and conjunctiva.

Atopic keratoconjunctivitis

    - Common in patients with atopy(ie: eczema, allergies, asthma, rhinitis)

Caustic keratoconjunctivitis

    - Secondary to chemical orbital exposure

Epidemic keratoconjunctivitis

- Highly contagious viral(Adenovirus) conjunctivitis, associated with watery discharge

Ultraviolet keratitis

- Secondary to UV light exposure

Keratoconjunctivitis sicca

- Associated with autoimmune disorders such as Sjogren's Syndrome, Sarcoidosis, Rheumatoid arthritis, and Scleroderma

DIPLOPIA

Monocular Diplopia

- Double vision that persists when one eye is closed
- Related to intrinsic eye problem
- **Differential Diagnosis**
    - Cataract
    - Lens Dislocation
    - Macular Disruption

Binocular Diplopia

- Double vision that resolves when the other eye is closed
- Related to a problem with visual axis alignment
- **3 Main Causes Binocular Diplopia**
    - Eye Musculature Dysfunction
    - Cranial Nerve Dysfunction
    - Brainstem or Intracranial process
- **Differential Diagnosis**
    - Basilar Artery Thrombosis
    - Posterior Communicating Artery (PCOM) Aneurysm
    - Vertebral Artery Dissection
    - Myasthenia Gravis
    - Lambert-Eaton Syndrome
    - Botulism

- Cavernous Sinus Thrombosis
- Brainstem Mass
- Intracranial Mass
- Miller Fischer variant Guillain-Barré
- MS
- Hyperthroid Proptosis
- Basilar Meningitis
- CVA
- Muscular Entrapment from Trauma
- Third nerve palsy
- Evaluation with CT/CTA to rule out a compressive mass or aneurysm

CENTRAL RETINAL ARTERY & VEIN OCCLUSION

- Restoration of blood flow within 100min may lead to complete recovery
- Occlusion >240min leads to irreversible damage
- **Etiology includes**
    - Embolism
    - Thrombosis (Hypercoagulable states)
    - Temporal Arteritis
    - Vasculitis
    - Sickle Cell Disease
    - Trauma
    - Vasospasm (migraine)
    - Glaucoma
    - Low retinal blood flow (carotid stenosis or hypotension)
- Consult ophthalmology with goals for reducing intraocular pressure, dislodging the embolus or increasing arterial flow
- Start high dose systemic corticosteroids if high ESR/CRP and sudden vision loss

UV KERATITIS

- Common conditions include photokeratitis, welder's flash, or snow blindness
- Caused by a lack of proper eye protection with prolonged UV exposure
- Eye exam (including slit lamp) may show:
  - Surrounding eyelid and face may appear mildly erythematous and edematous (consistent with sunburn)
  - Obvious tearing, discomfort, blepharospasm on exam with relief of symptoms after instilling topical anesthetic
  - **Fluorescein exam - Superficial Punctate Keratitis - small, pinpoint areas of increased uptake on cornea**

CONJUNCTIVITIS

Newborn

- Azithromycin 20mg/kg PO once daily for 3 days or
- Erythromycin 12.5 mg/kg PO q6hrs for 14 days

Chlamydial

- Doxycycline 100mg BID for 7 days or
- Azithromycin 1g (20mg/kg) PO one time dose

Gonococcal

- Ceftriaxone 1g IM one dose and

Bacterial Conjunctivitis

- Polymyxin B/Trimethoprim (Polytrim) 2 drops every 6 hours for 7 days or
- Erythromycin applied to the conjunctiva q6hrs fir 7 days or
- Levofloxacin 0.5% ophthalmic solution 1-2 drops every 2 hours for 2 days THEN every 6 hours for 5 days or
- Moxifloxacin 0.5% ophthalmic 1-2 drops every 2 hours for 2 days THEN every 6 hours for 5 days or
- Azithromycin 1% ophthalmic solution 1 drop BID for 2 days THEN 1 drop daily for 5 days

ACUTE ANGLE-CLOSURE GLAUCOMA

- Obstructed aqueous outflow tract → aqueous humor builds up → increased intraocular pressure (IOP) → optic nerve damage → vision loss
- **Increased posterior chamber pressure causes iris to bulge forward (iris bombé) causes further obstruction of outflow tract and causes further increase IOP**
- Acute attack is usually precipitated by pupillary dilation
- **At least 3 of these signs:**
    - IOP >21 mm Hg
    - Conjunctival injection
    - Corneal epithelial edema
    - Mid-dilated nonreactive pupil
    - Shallow anterior chamber with occlusion
- **At least 2 of these symptoms:**
    - Ocular pain
    - Nausea/vomiting
    - History of intermittent blurring of vision with halos

Decrease production of aqueous humor

- **Timolol 0.5%:**
    - Blocks beta receptors on ciliary epithelium
    - 1 drop in affected eye, repeat in 1 hour if needed.
- **Acetazolamide:**
    - Blocks productions of HCO_3^-, which draws Na^+ into the eye; water follows by osmosis to form aqueous humour
    - 500mg IV or PO (PO preferred unless patient is nauseated)
    - Can substitute methazolamide 100mg if patient has renal failure.
    - Contraindicated in sickle cell patients
- **Dorzolamide (Trusopt) 2%:**
    - topical carbonic anhydrase inhibitor
    - 1 drop in affected eye

α2 agonist

- **Brimonidine ophthalmic (alphagan) 0.2% OR Apraclonidine ophthalmic 1%:**

- α agonist will increase trabecular outflow
- 1 drop in affected eye

Facilitate outflow of aqueous humor

- **Pilocarpine 1%–2%:**
  - Parasympatholytic alkaloid acts on muscarinic receptors found on iris sphincter muscle → causes muscle to contract → miosis → pulls iris away from trabecular network
  - 1 drop in affected eye every 15 minutes x 2-4 doses, then every 4 to 6 hours
- Likely does not work until IOP drops below 40-50 mmHg, but still give immediately upon diagnosis
- Note: may make fundoscopic evaluation more difficult for ophtho consultant due to miosis

Reduce volume of aqueous humor

- These therapies are usually resolved for failure of other treatments. Hyper osmotic agents such as mannitol are effective but are contraindicated in renal failure and can cause hypotension in the volume depleted patient.
  - Mannitol: 1-2 g/kg IV given over 45 minutes to minimize cerebral effects (most common)

HYPHEMA

- Grossly visible blood in the anterior chamber of the eye

Causes

- Ocular trauma
- **Spontaneous hyphema (non-traumatic hyphema)**
  - Sickle cell disease
  - Ocular or laser surgery
  - HSV, VZV uveitis
  - Malignancy

Treatment

- Elevate head of bed and upright position to layer blood by gravity, open visual field while blood resorbs
- If IOP elevated (>22) the treatment is similar to glaucoma management except if there is also a concern for a retrobulbar hematoma as a result of trauma. Topical and oral treatments include
    - Timolol
    - Topical α-adrenergic agonist
    - Carbonic anhydrase inhibitors

HYPOPYON

- It is a leukocytic exudate seen in the anterior chamber
- A sign of inflammation of the anterior uvea and iris, i
- The exudate settles at the dependent aspect of the eye due to gravity
- **Differential**
    - Corneal ulcer
    - Behcet's disease
    - Endophthalmitis
- Requires emergent ophtho consult

ENDOPHTHALMITIS

- Inflammation (usually infectious) of the deep eye structures (aqueous and vitreus chambers)
- Staphylococcus, Streptococcus, Bacillus cereus
- Frequently leads to loss of vision
- Often associated with an open globe due to the invasive organism

UVEITIS

- Uveitis is inflammation of iris, ciliary body, and/or choroid
- **Anterior uveitis**
    - Topical steroid (anterior only; typically in consultation with ophthalmology)
    - Mydriatics (sympathomimetics)
    - Cycloplegics relieve pain

OPTIC NEURITIS

- Inflammatory, demyelinating condition of the optic nerve highly associated with MS
- 50% will go on to develop MS
- Acute, usually monocular, vision loss occurring over days (occasionally over hours)
- MRI of brain and orbits with gadolinium is necessary for diagnosis

RETINAL DETACHMENT

Types of detachment include

- **Rhegmatogenous (rhegma means "tear")**
    - As vitreous separates from retina the traction creates a hole in retina
    - Fluid goes through the hole and peels the retina off like wallpaper
- **Exudative**
    - Fluid accumulates beneath the retina without a retinal tear
    - Associated with neoplasm, inflammatory conditions, hypertension, preeclampsia
- **Tractional**
    - Acquired fibrocellular bands in the vitrous contract and detach the retina
    - Associated with DM, sickle cell, trauma
- **Distinguish between mac-off and mac-on with ultrasound**
- Requires emergent ophthalmology consult

Orthopedics

DIABETIC FOOT INFECTION

- Associated organisms include Staphylococcus, Streptococcus, Enterococcus, Enterobacteriaceae, Proteus, Bacteroides, and Pseudomonas, and Klebsiella

Mild-Moderate

- Clindamycin 450mg PO q8hrs daily x 14 days or
- TMP/SMX 2DS tabs PO q12hrs daily x 14 days or
- Doxycycline 100mg PO q12hrs daily x 14 days

Severe

- Vancomycin 15-20mg/kg IV q12hrs plus
- Ampicillin/Sulbactam 3g IV q6hrs or
- Piperacillin/Tazobactam 4.5g IV q8hrs or
- Cefepime 2g IV q12hrs or

DISKITIS OR OSTEOMYELITIS

- Treatment targets S. aureus, Streptococcus, Pseudomonas, E. coli

Inpatient Therapy

- Vancomycin 15-20 mg/kg IV BID and:
    - Ceftriaxone 2g IV daily or
    - Cefepime 2g IV IV three times daily or
    - Ceftazidime 2g IV three times daily or
    - Ciprofloxacin 400mg IV three times daily

FELON

- Definitive treatment is drainage but antibiotic coverage for S. aureus and Strep (also consider herpetic whitlow prior to I&D)
    - Cephalexin 500mg PO q6hrs daily x 7 days or
    - TMP/SMX 2 DS tablets PO q12hrs x 7 days or
    - Clindamycin 450mg PO q8hrs x 7 days

OPEN FRACTURES

Gustillo-Anderson grading scale

- Open fractures can be classified using the Gustillo-Anderson grading scale
- As the grade increase, so does the risk of infection
- Grading is based on wound size, neurovascular injury, and contamination

Grade I
- Wound <1cm
- Little soft tissue injury or crush injury
- Moderately clean puncture site
- Infection risk 0-12%

- **Grade II**
- Laceration >1cm
- No extensive soft tissue damage, but slight or moderate crush injury
- Moderate contamination
- Infection risk 2-12%

- **Grade III**
    - Extensive damage to soft tissue, including neurovascular structures and muscle
    - High degree of contamination
    - Infection risk 5-50%
    - Further subcategorized:
    - III A: Fracture covered by soft tissue (Infection risk 5-10%)
    - III B: Loss of soft tissue and evidence of bone stripping (Infection risk 10-50%)
    - III C: Any fracture with an associated arterial injury that requires surgical repair (Infection risk 25-50%)

Prophylactic antibiotics for open fractures

Initiate as soon as possible; increased infection rate when delayed for >3 hours from injury (NNT 12.5)

- **Grade I & II Fractures Options**
    - 1st generation cephalosporin: e.g. Cefazolin (Ancef) 2g IV TID

- Allergy to above: Clindamycin or vancomycin (25mg/kg) IV
- **Grade III Fracture Options**
  - Treatment as above for Grade I/II
  - PLUS aminoglycoside: e.g. Gentamicin 300 mg (1-1.7mg/kg) IV
  - Once daily dosing has been shown to be safe and effective
  - Special Considerations
  - Concern for Clostridium (soil contamination, farm injuries, possible bowel contamination): single drug regimen of Piperacillin/Tazobactam 4.5g (80mg/kg) IV TID
  - Fresh water wounds: fluoroquinolones OR 3rd/4th generation cephalosporin
  - Saltwater wounds: doxycycline + ceftazidime OR fluoroquinolone

BOXER'S FRACTURE

- Fracture of the 4th or 5th metacarpal caused by an axial load, typically from punching a person or object
- Angulation >30° in the 4th digit or >40° in the 5th digit should be reduced
- **Splint in an ulnar gutter splint or with a forearm volar splint with extension over the head of the MCP**

MALLET FINGER

- Rupture of extensor tendon in area of distal phalanx distal to DIP joint
- May be accompanied by avulsion fracture
- Caused by forced flexion of extended DIP joint
- If untreated, leads to swan neck deformity
- Splint DIP joint in continuous slight hyperextension x 6 wk

JERSEY FINGER

- Avulsion of flexor tendon from distal phalanx
- Occurs from forced extension of flexed DIP (historically from grabbing someone's jersey with the tip of a finger)
- Finger splint in slight flexion at DIP

TRIGGER FINGER

- Tenosynovitis of the flexor sheath of the finger or thumb as a result of repetitive use
- Also known as stenosing tenosynovitis and is generally managed with NSAIDS

DE QUERVAIN TENOSYNOVITIS

- Tenosynovitis of abductor pollicis longus (APL), extensor pollicis brevis (EPB)
- Pain along radial aspect of wrist (may radiate to thumb or extend into the forearm)
- Splint thumb and wrist with daily range of motion exercises with NSAIDS for pain

GAMEKEEPER'S THUMB

- Ulnar collateral ligament ruptures at insertion into proximal phalanx (due to radial deviation of MCP)
- If left untreated, it will causes decreased thumb adduction and inability to perform opposition.
- The mechanism of injury is usually a rapid deceleration while holding onto an object (such as a ski pole)
- Compare relative laxity to other thumb.
- >35 degrees of joint laxity or 15 degrees of relative laxity compared to other thumb is diagnostic of a complete UCL rupture

DRUMMER'S WRIST

- Tenosynovitis of the 3rd dorsal wrist compartment containing the extensor pollicis longus (EPL)
- Classically drummers who play for long periods of time without rest

GANGLION CYST

- Cystic collection of synovial fluid within a joint or tendon sheath (most resolve spontaneously) and pain is treated with NSAIDS.

LUNATE FRACTURE

- A rare injury that also occurs via a FOOSH (fall on outstretched hand)
- Treat with a thumb spica splint

TRIQUETRUM FRACTURE

- 3rd most common carpal bone injury (following scaphoid and lunate fractures
- Treat with a wrist splint (forearm volar splint)

PISIFORM FRACTURE

- Occurs via fall onto hypothenar eminence
- Treat with compression dressing or forearm volar splint in 30 degrees of flexion with ulnar deviation

HAMATE FRACTURE

Hook (common)

- Associated with interrupted swing of club, bat, or racquet (handle impacts hypothenar eminence)
    - Compression dressing or Forearm volar splint
    - Nonunion is common and excision of bone may be necessary

Body (rare)

- Associated with fracture-dislocations of 4th/5th metacarpals
    - Stable: Forearm volar splint immobilization
    - Unstable (displaced, Guyon canal injury): splint immobilization and ortho referral

HIGH-PRESSURE INJECTION INJURY

- Surgical emergency (amputation rates are as high as 30%)
- Occurs with grease, paint, and fuel guns; usually injected into non-dominant hand
- Most important factor is type of injected material

GOUT AND PSEUDOGOUT

- Presence of crystals does not exclude septic arthritis
- The most important test on an arthrocentesis is the gram stain while awaiting culture, to rule out the presence of bacteria
    - Gout and Pseudogout should have NO bacterial on gram stain
- **Serum uric acid levels are not helpful (30% of patients with gout attack have normal levels)**

Crystalline analysis

- Gout: yellow monosodium urate; negatively birefringent; needle-shaped
- Pseudogout: calcium pyrophosphate; positively birefringent; rhomboid-shaped

Treatment

- **NSAID options include ibuprofen, naproxen and indomethacin**
- **Cochicine Can be used as alternative agent to NSAIDs in patient with normal renal/hepatic function**
    - 1.2mg PO (load), followed by 0.6mg one hour later x 1 (max 3 doses)
- **Prednisone 30-59mg PO x 5 days also provides substantial pain relief (caution in diabetic patients)**

ARTHROCENTESIS RESULTS AND DIAGNOSIS

	Normal	Noninflammatory	Inflammatory	Septic
Clarity	Transparent	Transparent	Cloudy	Cloudy
Color	Clear	Yellow	Yellow	Yellow
WBC	<200	<200-2000	200-50,000	>1,100 (prosthetic joint) >25,000; LR=2.9 >50,000; LR=7.7 >100,000; LR=28
PMN	<25%	<25%	>50%	>64% (prosthetic joint) >90%
Culture	Neg	Neg	Neg	>50% positive
Lactate	<5.6 mmol/L	<5.6 mmol/L	<5.6 mmol/L	>5.6 mmol/L

LDH	<250	<250	<250	>250
Crystals	None	None	Multiple or none	None

LUNOTRIQUETRAL LIGAMENT INSTABILITY

- Ulnar equivalent of the scapholunate ligament injury
- May be confused with other causes of ulnar-sided wrist pain
- Results from FOOSH with impact on hypothenar eminence
- X-ray can show wWidening of the triquetrolunate joint space
- Lunate tilts palmar producing zigzag pattern (opposite of scapholunate injury)

SCAPHOID FRACTURE

- Most commonly fractured carpal bone
- All patients with clinical suspicion should be treated regardless of X-ray findings
- X-ray - obtain both standard and scaphoid views
- Refer to a hand surgeon because may lead to osteonecrosis if not properly recognized/treated
- 25% of those with initially neg X-ray will actually have a fracture (typically found on delay X-ray or other modality)

NURSEMAID'S ELBOW

- Radial head subluxation due to longitudinal traction on arm as a result of the annular ligament of the radius displaces
- Generally in age 1-5yo
- Hyperpronation has greater first attempt success (94% vs 69%) compared to supination, although both have a similar reduction rate

Hyperpronation Technique

- Hold patient's elbow at 90 degrees with one hand
    - Place thumb over radial head to facilitate reduction and provide tactile feedback
- With other hand hyperpronate patient's wrist

Supination Technique

- Hold patient's elbow at 90 degrees with one hand
  - Place thumb over radial head to facilitate reduction and provide tactile feedback
- With other hand supinate patient's wrist and fully flex elbow

SUPRACONDYLAR FRACTURE

- Most common elbow fracture in patients age <8yr
- **Lateral and AP radiographs are usually sufficient, and in many instances demonstrate an obvious fracture. Often, however, no fracture line can be identified. In such cases assessing for indirect signs is essential:**
  - **Anterior fat pad sign (sail sign)**: the anterior fat pad is elevated by a joint effusion and appears as a lucent triangle on the lateral projection
  - **Posterior fat pad sign**
  - **Anterior humeral** line should intersect the middle third of the capitellum in most children although, in children under 4, the anterior humeral line may pass through the anterior third without injury

SALTER-HARRIS FRACTURES

- **S** 1 - Slipped (through physis/growth plate)
- **A** 2 - Above (physis with metaphysis fracture)
- **L** 3 - Lower (physis with epiphysis fracture)
- **T** 4 - Through (physis, metaphysis and epiphysis fracture)
- **R** 5 - Rammed (growth plate crushed)

Type	I (Slip)	II (Above)	III (Below)	IV (Through)	V (Crush)
Fracture Location	hypertrophic zone of physis (epiphysis separates from metaphysis)	Through physis and out through piece of metaphyseal bone	Intra-articular	Starts at articular surface and extends through epiphysis, physis, metaphysis	Physis compression

Pathophysiology	Growing cells remain on the epiphysis in continuity with blood supply	Growing cells remain on the epiphysis in continuity with blood supply	fracture extends from epiphysis through physis		
Epidemiology	Occurs mostly in infants and toddlers	Most common type of fracture			Typically occurs at knee or ankle
Prognosis	Good	Good	Moderate	Moderate	Highest chance of growth arrest

Pediatrics

PEDIATRIC ANTIBIOTICS

Pediatric fever of uncertain source (90 days - 36 months)

- Ceftriaxone (50-100mg/kg) and
- Consider vancomycin (15mg/kg)

Pediatric fever of uncertain source Neonates (up to 1 month of age)

- MRSA is uncommon in the neonate
- Ampicillin 50mg/kg IV q6hrs and
- Cefotaxime 50mg/kg IV q6hrs or Gentamicin 2.5mg/kg IV q8hrs
- If suspecting S. pneumoniae or MRSA, add Vancomycin
- Consider acyclovir for HSV

Pediatric fever of uncertain source > 1 month old

- Ceftriaxone 2gm (50mg/kg) IV BID daily and
- Vancomycin 15-20 mg/kg IV BID daily
- Vancomycin is for resistant Pneumococcus

VP shunt infections

- Empiric therapy: Vancomycin and Cefotaxime 200 mg/kg/day IV div Q6 or ceftriaxone 100 mg/kg/day IV div Q12-24
- Always consult neurosurgery if suspicious of a VP shunt

Mastoiditis, acute

- S. pneumo, S. pyogenes, S. aureus, H. flu, P. aeruginosa R/O meningitis.
- Surgical debridement as indicated.
- Ampicillin-Sulbactam (Unasyn) 300mg/kg/dau IV div Q6 or
- Cefotaxime 150mg/kg/day div Q8 or
- Ceftriaxone 50mg/kg/day Q24 or
- Clindamycin 40mg/kg/day IV div Q6 or vancomycin x21 days.

Conjunctivitis

- Highly contagious and artificial tears may help with symptoms.
- NEVER administer steroids.
- HSV types 1-2
- Polymyxin/trimethoprim ophthalmic solution 1 drop Q3 x 7-10 days

Dacryocystitis

- Warm compresses and tear duct massage. Antibiotics are often not needed

Orbital Cellulitis

- Ampicillin-Sulbactam (Unasyn) 300mg/kg/day IV div Q6 or
- Cefotaxime 150mg/kg/day div Q8 or
- Ceftriaxone 50mg/kg/day Q24 and Nafcillin 200mg/kg/day IV div Q6.

Periorbital (preseptal) Cellulitis

- Nafcillin 200mg/kg/day IV div Q6 or
- Cefazolin 100mg/kg/day IV Q8 x7-10 days.
- If MRSA suspected, Vancomycin or Clindamycin 40mg/kg/day IV div Q6.

Otitis Externa

- Clean canal often.
- Neomycin/Polymyxin B and/or hydrocortisone otic drops or
- Ofloxacin or Ciprofloxacin solution.

Ludwig's Angina

- **Immunocompetent:**
  - Ampicillin/Sulbactam 3g (50mg/kg) IV q6 hrs or
  - Penicillin G 2-4 million units IV q6 hrs + Metronidazole 500 mg IV q6 hrs or
  - Clindamycin 600 mg IV q6 hrs (option for those allergic to penicillin)
- **Immunocompromised**
  - Cefepime 2 g IV q12 hrs + Metronidazole 500 mg IV q6 hrs or
  - Meropenem 1 g IV q8 hrs or
  - Imipenem/Cilastatin 500mg (20mg/kg) IV q6 hours or

- Piperacillin-tazobactam 4.5g (80mg/kg) IV q6 hours

Dental abscess

- Clindamycin 40mg/kg/day PO/IV/IM div Q6 or Penicillin G 100,000-200,000 U/kg/day IV div Q6.

Gingivostomatitis

- Acyclovir PO 80mg/kg/day div Q6 x7 days.

Bacterial tracheitis

- Third generation cephalosporin (cefotaxime or ceftriaxone) plus
- MRSA coverage, options below depending on prevalence of MRSA
  - Clindamycin 40mg/kg/d IV divided q8hr or
  - Vancomycin 45mg/kg/d IV divided q8hr

Epiglottitis

- Cefotaxime 150mg/kg/day div Q8 or
- Ceftriaxone 50mg/kg/day Q24.

Pharyngitis

- Perform a throat culture before treating.
  - Penicillin V 25-50mg/kg/day PO div TID-QID or Amoxicillin 50-75mg/kg/day div BID-TID x10 days or
  - Penicillin G Benzathine 600,000 U IM (<27 kg), 1.2 million U (>27 kg) x1 or
  - Erythromycin or Clindamycin for PCN-allergic patients.

Pneumonia

- Coverage targeted at S. pneumoniae, H. influenzae. M. pneumoniae, C. pneumoniae, and Legionella (elderly)

- **1-3 Month**
- Hospitalized
- Afebrile pneumonitis
- Erythromycin (10 mg/kg q6) or azithro (2.5 mg/kg q12)
- Febrile pneumonia

- Add cefoTAXime (200mg/kg per day divided q8h)
- Outpatient
- erythromycin or azithro PO

>3mo - 18 years

- Hospitalized (PICU/severely ill)
- Ceftriaxone IV and vancomycin and consider azithromycin
- Hospitalized (moderately ill)
- Fully immunized: Ampicillin (50mg/kg q6) IV
- Not fully immunized: Ceftriaxone IV
- Outpatient
- Amoxicillin (90 mg/kg divided BID) x 5 days PO
- Alternative: clindamycin or azithromycin or amoxicillin-clavulanate

Pertussis

- **< 1 month old**
  - Same antibiotics for active disease and post-exposure prophylaxis
  - Azithromycin 10mg/kg (max 500mg/day) daily x 5 days
- **>1 month old**
  - Azithromycin 10mg/kg (max 500mg/day) daily x 5 days
  - if > 6 months old then day 2-5 of treatment should be reduced to 5mg/kg (250mg/day max)
  - TMP/SMX 4mg/kg PO BID daily for 14 days (if > 2 months old)
- **Adults**
  - Azithromycin 500mg PO once daily for day #1 then 250mg PO once daily for days #2-5 or
  - Clarithromycin 500mg BID x7 days or
  - Erythromycin 500mg QID x7 days

Endocarditis

- **Dental prophylaxis indicated for prosthetic cardiac valves or valvular repair or prosthetic material used for cardiac valve repair.**
- Previous infectious endocarditis.
- Congenital heart disease (CHD) - except for the conditions listed below, antibiotic prophylaxis is no longer recommended for any other form of CHD.

- Unrepaired cyanotic CHD, including palliative shunts and conduits.
- Completely repaired CHD with prosthetic material or device, whether placed by surgery or by catheter intervention, during the first 6 months after the procedure.
- Repaired CHD with residual defects at the site or adjacent to the site or a prosthetic patch or prosthetic device (which inhibit endotheliazation).
- Cardiac transplantation recipients who develop cardiac valvulopathy.
- **Prophylaxis for oral, dental, respiratory tract or high risk patients with chronic GI/GU infections**
- Amoxicillin 50mg/kg PO x1 or Ampicillin 50mg/kg IV x1, 30-60 minutes prior to the procedure.
- Allergic patients: Clindamycin 20mg/kg PO/IV x1 or cephalexin 50mg/kg PO x1 or Azithromycin 15mg/kg PO x1.
- **Empiric therapy, native valves: S. viridnas, Enterococci, Staphylococci**
- By definition includes multiple positive blood cultures, new murmur of valvular insufficiency, emboli and echo evidence of vegetations. Send cultures and target therapy based on results. Vancomycin and Gentamicin pending culture results.

UTI

- **Inpatient:**
- >2 months: Cefotaxime or Ceftriaxone until taking PO, well appearing → transition to outpatient therapy.
- **Outpatient: (Infants and Children):**
- TMP-SMX (Bactrim) 6-10mg/kg/day TMP component div BID or Cefixime 16mg/kg/day x1 day, then 8mg/kg/day Q24 (max 400mg/dose) or Cephalexin 25mg/kg/dose QID (max 1000mg/dose) x7-14 days. Alternatives: Nitrofurantoin, Ciprofloxacin, Ceftriaxone. (Adults): Bactrim DS BID x3 days or Ciprofloxacin 250mg BID x3 days.
- Skin & Soft Tissue Infections

Skin abscess

- OSSA/MSSA - Cephalexin 50-75mg/kg/day PO div TID or Augmentin 80-90mg/kg/day PO div BID x5-7 days. I&D when indicated.
- If MRSA prevalent or if recurrent abscess, send specimen for culture and sensitivity. Treat with Clindamycin 40mg/kg/day IV div Q6 or TMP-

SMX (Bactrim) 5mg/kg/dose TMP Q6-8. If toxic-appearing, use vancomycin.

Cellulitis

- Start IV: Clindamycin 40mg/kg/day IV div Q6 if high community incidence of MRSA. May use Nafcillin 200mg/kg/day IV div Q6 or Cefazolin 100mg/kg/day IV div Q8 if low incidence of MRSA. Transition to PO when stable. If no improvement, change to Vancomycin (dose by age).
- PO: Cephalexin 50-75mg/kg/day divided TID or Dicloxacillin 50mg/kg/day PO div Q6. Total duration of treatment 7-10 days.

Erysipelas

- Penicillin G IV, then transition to Penicillin V or Amoxicillin PO;x10 days.

Impetigo

- Mupirocin topical to lesions TID, cleanse with soap and water. Bathe daily. If extensive, treat with Cephalexin PO or Amoxicillin-Clavunate x5-7 days.

Omphalitis/Funisitis

- Empiric: Cefotaxime and Clindamycin x10 or more days. If MRSA prevalent, Amoxicillin, Cephalexin.
- Funisitis (local infection of cord): cord care, topical antimicrobials.

Paronychia

- Local wound care and I&D unless signs of spreading infection, then consider Augmentin or Clindamycin.

Scabies

- Topical 5% Permethrin cream, apply to neck down, wash off in 8-14 hours.
- Topical Lindane 1%, 1 oz lotion/30 g cream, apply to neck down, wash off in 8 hours.

Staph scaled skin syndrome

- Nafcillin 200mg/kg/day IV div Q6 or Cefazolin IV x5-7 days. Consider vancomycin.

Tinea corporis

- May use one of many topical anti-fungal agents:
    - Terbinafine 1% cream or gel BID to affected areas or
    - Clotrimazole 1% cream, lotion or solution;

Tinea capitis

- Griseofulvin 10-20mg/kg/day div Q12-24 (max 1000mg/day) or
- Griseofulvin >2 years 5-10mg/kg/day div Q12-24 x6 weeks] and Selenium sulfide shampoo twice weekly x1 week as directed.

Pulmonology

ARDS

- Non-cardiogenic pulmonary edema due to lung capillary endothelial injury (diffuse alveolar damage)
- New onset respiratory symptoms
- Bilateral pulmonary opacities
- Symptoms not explained by cardiac etiology or volume overload
- Ventilator Settings
- Permissive hypercapnia
- Tidal volume 6-8cc/kg of predicted body weight
    - Limit barotrauma to healthy area of lung
    - Increase PEEP to improve oxygenation

ASTHMA

- Reversible airway obstruction
- Chest X-ray rarely needed unless suspicion of an infectious etiology or pneumothorax

Albuterol

- Intermittent: 2.5-5mg q20min x3, then 2.5-10mg q1-4hr as needed or continuous: 0.5mg/kg/hr (max 15mg/hr)

Ipratropium

- 0.25-0.5mg q20min x2-3 doses

Steroids

- Dexamethasone effective as other steroids especially in children and most likely adults as well (0.6mg/kg IV or PO max 16mg)
- Methylprednisolone: 1mg/kg IV q 4–6hr (only use IV if cannot tolerate PO)
- Prednisone 40-60mg/day = for adults one x5 doses

Magnesium

- 25-75 mg/kg over 30 min (1-2 gm IV in most adults) decreased rate of admission for moderate to severe asthma

Epinephrine

- 1:1000 0.01 mg/kg (max 0.5mg) IM Q20min x3

Non-invasive ventilation

- Alleviates muscle fatigue which leads to larger tidal volumes
- may drive nebulized treatments deeper into airways
- Also maximize inspiratory support

COPD

- Airflow obstruction that is not fully reversible (as compared to asthma)
- **Treatment mirrors asthma therapies except lack of similar efficacy from magnesium**

Antibiotics options

- Indicated for patients with purulent sputum or
- Increased sputum production or
- Requiring non invasive positive pressure ventilation
    - Azithromycin 500mg PO BID or
    - Doxycycline 100mg PO BID or
    - Levofloxacin 500mg PO BID

PULMONARY HYPERTENSION

- Since right ventricle is dependent on preload, RV contractility and afterload, severe pulmonary arterial hypertension causes pathological changes to right ventricle
- Finding may or may not include:
    - Elevated BNP
    - ECG findings (similar to acute pulmonary embolism):
        - Right axis deviation
        - Evidence of right heart strain on bedside ultrasound or CT
        - S1Q3T3 ECG finding

- T-wave inversions on ECG in inferior and anteroseptal leads
- Right ventricular hypertrophy
- Large R waves in precordial leads
- Tachyarrhythmias

Optimize (usually reduce) RV preload

- Usually euvolemic or hypervolemic, rarely need IV fluids so diuretics can benefit and treat the RV failure

Increase cardiac output

- Vasopressors can augment MAP >65 mmHg and then start low dose dobutamine (5-10mcg/kg/min)

Reduce RV afterload

- Focus on correcting hypoxia which will dilate a pulmonary artery

Treat arrhythmias

Adjunctive Chronic therapies

- Prostacyclin (vasodilatation, inhibit platelet aggregation)
- Phosphodiesterase Type 5 (PDE5) Inhibitors (vasodilation, increases RV contractility)
- Endothelin receptor antagonists (vasodilation)

DROWNING

- Hypoxemia due to aspiration
- Cerebral edema and elevated ICP from prolonged hypoxia
- Hypoxemia and hypothermia cause arrhythmias (VF/VT)
- Respiratory / metabolic acidosis
- Hypothermia from even short submersions
- Observe for 6 hours and only consider discharge if hemodynamically stable, with no hypoxia, and normal CXR - otherwise admit for observation

FOREIGN BODY ASPIRATION

- CXR is normal in > 50% of patients

- Patients require CT and/or bronchoscopy for definitive diagnosis and removal

HEMOPTYSIS

- Nebulized TXA 0.5g
- Intubate with >8.0
- If possible can selectively intubate the unaffected bronchus to prevent aspiration
- Placing patient with affected lung down may actually worsen V-Q mismatch
- Correct any coagulopathy

HEMOPTYSIS DIFFERENTIAL DIAGNOSIS

Infectious

- Bronchitis
- PNA
- Lung abscess
- TB
- Plague

Neoplastic

- Lung cancer
- Metastatic cancer

Cardiovascular

- PE
- CHF
- Pulmonary HTN
- AV malformation
- Mitral stenosis

Alveolar hemorrhage syndromes

- Goodpasture
- Wegener

- SLE

Hematologic

- Uremia
- Platelet dysfunction (ASA, clopidogrel)
- Anticoagulant therapy

Traumatic

- Foreign body aspiration
- Ruptured bronchus

Inflammatory

- Bronchiectasis
- Cystic Fibrosis
- Cocaine inhalation (crack lung)
- Goodpasture syndrome

MEDIASTINITIS AND PNEUMOMEDIASTINUM

- Commonly caused by esophageal rupture or perforation
- Infection may be caused by esophageal rupture/perforation or spread of infection from remote site
- Other etiologies can include
    - Prior cardiovascular surgery
    - Esophageal rupture (Boerhaave Syndrome)
    - Ludwig Angina
    - Thoracic Trauma
    - Lung infection extensionStreptococcus and Bacteroides

PNEUMOTHORAX

Tension pneumothorax

- Causes obstructive shock by preventing venous return to the right side of the heart

Spontaneous pneumothorax

- Can primary or secondary due to an underlying structural abnormality such as with COPD/Asthma or a malignancy

Catamenial pneumothorax

- Spontaneous, recurrent pneumothorax in women of reproductive age, associated with menses

Traumatic pneumothorax

Iatrogenic pneumothorax

PULMONARY EMBOLISM (PE)

- Only 40% of ambulatory ED patients with PE have concomitant DVT

Massive

- Causes a cardiac arrest or sustained hypotension

Submassive

- RV dysfunction (RV dilation) or elevated troponin but without hypotensive
- ECG can show a new complete or incomplete RBBB, anteroseptal ST elevation/depression or TWI

Sub-Segmental

- Limited to the sub-segmental pulmonary arteries

PNEUMONIA

Risk Factor	Associated Organism
COPD	• S. pneumoniae • Haemophilus influenzae • Moraxella • Legionella

Healthcare associated	• S. pneumoniae • Gram-negative bacilli • H. influenzae • Staphylococcus aureus • Anaerobes • Chlamydophila pneumoniae
Exposure to bird droppings	Histoplasma capsulatum
Exposure to birds	Chlamoydophila psittaci
Exposure to rabbits	Francisella tularensis
Exposure to farm animals	Coxiella burnetii (Q fever)
Exposure to southwestern US	Coccidiomycosis (Valley fever)
HIV	• S. pneumoniae • H. influenzae • M. tuberculosis • Pneumocystis jiroveci • Cryptococcus • Histoplasma
Aspiration	Anaerobes
Injection drug use	• S. aureus • Anaerobes • M. tuberculosis • S. Pneumo
Ventilator Associated Pneumonia	• Pseudomonas aeruginosa • Acinetobacter sp. • Stenotrophomonas maltophilia

TRACHEOSTOMY COMPLICATIONS

• If a patient with a trach. requires positive pressure ventilation, ensure the cuff is inflated

Tracheostomy obstruction

• Usually from mucous plug
• Remove inner cannula

Tracheostomy dislodgement

- Re-insert with neck hyperextended
- Use same size or next smaller size

Tracheostomy infection

- Tracheitis
- Antibiotics for Staph, Pseudomonas and Candida

Tracheostomy bleeding

- Local Bleeding
    - Inflate the balloon if cuffed trach.
- Tracheo-innominate artery fistula
    - Rare but life-threatening bleed
        - Usually 1-3 weeks post-op
        - Local digital pressure or hyper-inflate cuff

PNEUMONIA

- Double coverage for S. pneumoniae is increasingly required while single coverage for influenzae. M. pneumoniae, C. pneumoniae, and Legionella is acceptable

Healthy

- Azithromycin 500mg PO day 1, 250mg on days 2-5 or
- Doxycycline 100mg BID x 10-14d (2nd line choice) plus
    - Amoxicillin/Clavulanate 2g BID and

Unhealthy

- Chronic heart, lung, liver, or renal disease; DM, alcoholism, malignancy.
- Levofloxacin 750mg QD x5d or
- Moxifloxacin 400mg QD x7-14d or
- Amoxicillin/Clavulanate 2g BID and
- Azithromycin 500mg day 1, 250mg days 2-5 or
- Doxycycline 100mg PO BID x 7-10 days or
- Clarithromycin 500mg PO BID x 7-10 days

Inpatient

- Mono-therapy or combination therapy is acceptable. Combination therapy includes a cephalosporin and macrolide targeting atypicals and Strep Pneumonia 1]
- The use of adjunctive corticosteroids (methylprednisolone 0.5 mg/kg IV BID x 5d) in CAP of moderate-high severity (PSI Score IV or V; CURB-65 ≥ 2) is associated with:
- ↓ mortality (3%)
- ↓ need for mechanical ventilation (5%)
- ↓ length of hospital stay (1d)

Community Acquired (Non-ICU)

- Coverage against community acquired organisms plus M. catarrhalis, Klebsiella, S. aureus
- Levofloxacin 750mg IV/PO once daily or
- Moxifloxacin 400mg IV/PO once daily or
- Ceftriaxone 1g IV once daily and
- Azithromycin 500mg IV/PO once daily or
- Doxycycline 100mg IV/PO BID

Hospital Acquired or Ventilator Associated Pneumonia

- 3-drug regimen recommended options:
    - Cefepime 1-2gm q8-12h or ceftazidime 2gm q8h and Levofloxacin 750 mg PO/IV every 24 hours and Vancomycin 15mg/kg q12 or
    - Imipenem 500mg q6hr and cipro 400mg q8hr and vanco 15mg/kg q12 or
    - Piperacillin-Tazobactam 4.5gm q6h and cipro 400mg q8h and vanco 15mg/kg q12
    - Consider tobramycin in place of fluoroquinolones given FDA 2016 warnings

Ventilator Associated Pneumonia

- High Risk of MRSA: Use 3-Drug Regimen. Several options are available, but recommendation is to include an antibiotic from each of these categories:

- **MRSA Antibiotic:** Vancomycin 15mg/kg q12h or Linezolid 600 mg IV q12h and
- **Anti-pseudomonal Antibiotic:** Piperacillin-Tazobactam 4.5gm q6h or Cefepime 2 g IV q8h or Imipenem 500 mg IV q6h or Aztreonam 2 g IV q8h and
- **GN Antibiotic With Anti-pseudomonal Activity:** Cipro 400 mg IV q8h

ICU, low risk of pseudomonas

- Ceftriaxone 1gm IV and Azithromycin 500mg IV or
- Ceftriaxone 1gm IV and (moxifloxacin 400mg IV or levofloxacin 750mg IV)
- Penicillin allergy
- (Moxifloxacin or levofloxacin) and (aztreonam 1-2gm IV or clindamycin 600mg IV)

ICU, risk of pseudomonas

- Cefepime, Imipenem, or Piperacillin/Tazobactam and IV cipro/levo
- Cefepime, imipenem, or piperacillin-tazobactam and gent and azithromycin
- Cefepime, imipenem, or piperacillin-tazobactam and gent and cipro/levo

Psychiatry

SUICIDE

- Women attempt suicide more often; men complete more often.
- Suicide completion risk factors
- Prior suicide attempts
- Detailed suicide plan
- Access to weapons
- Age > 45
- Drug or alcohol use
- Psychiatric problems
- Lack of social support
- Male
- Recent emotional, financial or social stresses
- Terminal medical condition

CHEMICAL RESTRAINTS

- Ideal medication is IV, IM, and IN with a short half-life, rapid onset, and minimal respiratory depression.
- Haloperidol - Typical antipsychotic - adverse effect: QT prolongation - less commonly used prehospital.
- Benzodiazepines - Adverse effect: respiratory depression - can safely be combined with an antipsychotic.
- Ketamine - Emerging as an alternative but long duration can make hospital evaluation of the patient difficult. (4mg/kg IM or 1-2mg/kg IV)

RENAL

ACUTE RENAL FAILURE

Pre-renal

- **Hypovolemia**
  - GI: decreased intake, vomiting and diarrhea
  - Hemorrhage
  - Pharmacologic: diuretics
  - Third spacing
  - Pancreatitis
  - Skin losses: fever, burns
  - Miscellaneous
  - Hypoaldosteronism
  - Salt-losing nephropathy
  - Post-obstructive diuresis
- **Hypotension**
  - Sepsis
  - Decreased cardiac output
  - Hepatorenal Syndrome
    - Ischemia/infarction
    - Valvulopathy
  - Pharmacologic
    - Beta-blockers
    - Calcium-channel blockers
    - Antihypertensive medications
  - High output heart failure
    - Thyrotoxicosis
    - AV fistula
  - Renal artery and small-vessel disease
    - Embolism: thrombotic, septic, cholesterol
    - Thrombosis: atherosclerosis, vasculitis, sickle cell disease
    - Dissection

- Pharmacologic
- Microvascular thrombosis
  - Preeclampsia
  - Hemolytic Uremic Syndrome (HUS)
  - Thrombotic Thrombocytopenic Purpura (TTP)
  - Disseminated Intravascular Coagulation (DIC)
  - Vasculitis
  - Sickle Cell Disease
- Hypercalcemia

Intrinsic

- Tubular diseases
- Nephrotoxins
- Interstitial diseases
- Glomerular diseases
- Small-vessel diseases
- Abdominal compartment syndrome
- Hepatorenal syndrome
- Cardiorenal syndrome

Post-renal

- Urethra and bladder outlet
- Anatomic malformations
- Urethral atresia
- Meatal stenosis
- Anterior and posterior urethral valves
- Ureter
- Anatomic malformations
- Vesicoureteral reflux (female preponderance)
- Ureterovesical junction obstruction
- Ureterocele
- Retroperitoneal tumor
- Various locations in GU tract
- Trauma

- Blood clot
- Urethra and bladder outlet
- Phimosis or urethral stricture (male preponderance)
- Neurogenic bladder
- Diabetes mellitus, spinal cord disease, multiple sclerosis, Parkinson's
- Pharmacologic: anticholinergics, a-adrenergic antagonists, opioids
- Urethra and bladder outlet
- BPH
- Cancer of prostate, bladder, cervix, or colon
- Obstructed catheters
- Calculi, uric acid crystals
- Papillary necrosis
- Tumor: Ureter, uterus, prostate, bladder, colon, rectum; retroperitoneal lymphoma
- Retroperitoneal fibrosis: idiopathic, tuberculosis, sarcoidosis, propranolol
- Stricture: TB, radiation, schistosomiasis, NSAIDs
- Aortic aneurysm
- Pregnant uterus
- IBD
- Trauma

HYPOCALCEMIA

- Low <8.5 (<2.0 ionized)
- Low! <6.5 (<1.5 ionized)
- Correct for hypoalbuminemia
    - Corrected Ca = (0.8 *(Normal Alb - Patient's Alb)) + Serum Ca

Causes

- **Misc**
    - Shock
    - Sepsis

- Pancreatitis
- Hypomag
- Rhabdo (phosphate overload)
- Massive transfusion
- Systemic Hydrofluoric Acid toxicity
- DiGeorge syndrome
- **Decreased absorption**
  - Vitamin D deficiency
- **Increased excretion**
  - Alcoholism
  - Renal Failure
  - Diuretics
- **Endocrine**
  - Hypoparathyroidism
- **Drugs**
  - Cimetidine
  - Phenytoin
  - Lasix, loop diuretics
  - Norepinephrine
  - Glucagon
  - Glucocorticoids
  - Magnesium sulfate
  - Nitroprusside

ECG findings

- QT Prolongation via increasing the ST length
- Only hypothermia and hypocalcemia prolong QT this way

Treatment

- **Asymptomatic**
  - Calcium gluconate 1 gm PO Q6hrs
  - Vitamin D (calcitriol) 0.2 mcg BID
- **Symptomatic**
  - Calcium gluconate/chloride 10mL of 10% soln IV over 10min

- Correct hypomag at same time (otherwise PTH is inhibited)
- Avoid phenothiazine antipsychotics (may precipitate extrapyramidal symptoms)
- Avoid furosemide (may worsen hypocalcemia)

HYPERCALCEMIA

- High >10.5 meq/L (>2.7 ionized)
- High! >12.0 meq/L
- 90% of cases associated with malignancy or hyperparathyroidism
- Symptoms most correlated with rate of rise of Ca, not absolute level

Mnemonic: Stones, Bones, Groans, Moans, Thrones, Psychic Overtones

- **"Stones"**
    - Renal calculi
    - Renal failure
- **"Bones"**
    - Bone pain/destruction
- **"Groans"**
    - Abdominal pain, vomiting
    - Dehydration
    - Pancreatitis
- **"Thrones"**
    - Polyuria/polydipsia (Renal insufficiency)
    - Constipation
- **"Psychic Overtones"**
    - Lethargy/confusion/Hallucinations

Causes of Hypercalcemia

- Hypercalcemia of malignancy
- Hyperparathyroidism
- Lithium
- Thiazides
- Hypothyroidism
- Addison's

- Paget's
- Sarcoid
- Hyperthyroid
- Milk-alkali syndrome
- Excess vitamin D
- Calciphylaxis

Asymptomatic or Ca <12 mg/dL

- Does not require immediate treatment
- Advise to avoid factors that can aggravate hypercalcemia (thiazide diuretics, Li, volume depletion, prolonged inactivity, high Ca diet)

Mildly symptomatic Ca 12-14 mg/dL

- May not require immediate therapy; however, an acute rise may cause symptoms

Symptomatic or Severe hypercalcemia (Ca >14 mg/dL)

- Patients should be admitted for observation
- **Hydration**
    - Isotonic saline at 200-300 mL/hour; adjust to maintain urine output at 100-150 mL/hour
- **Calcitonin**
    - Consider adding calcitonin 4 units/kg SC or IV q12hr in patients w/ Ca >14 mg/dL (3.5 mmol/L) who are also symptomatic (lowers Ca w/in 2-4hr)
    - Tachyphylaxis limits use long term, but is a great choice for emergent cases
- **Bisphosphonates**
    - Give for severe hypercalcemia due to excessive bone resorption (lowers Ca within 12-48hr)
    - Pamidronate 90mg IV over 24 hours OR
    - Zoledronate 4mg IV over 15 minutes
- **Electrolyte Repletion**
    - Correct hypokalemia
    - Correct hypomagnesemia
- **Diuresis**

- Furosemide is NOT routinely recommended
- Only consider in patients with renal insufficiency or heart failure and volume overload

- **Dialysis**
  - Consider if patient:
  - Anuric with Renal Failure
  - Failing all other therapy
  - Severe hypervolemia not amenable to diuresis
  - Serum Calcium level >18mg/dL

- **Corticosteroids**
  - Decrease Ca mobilization from bone and are helpful with steroid-sensitive tumors (e.g. lymphoma, MM)
  - Prednisone 60mg PO daily

HYPERPHOSPHATEMIA

Causes

- Increased phosphate intake (Vitamin D, laxative abuse)
- Increased renal reabsorption (Hypoparathyroidism)
- Decreased excretion (Renal failure
- Transcellular shifts (Tumor lysis syndrome, Rhabdomyolysis)

Differential Diagnosis

- Calciphylaxis
- Vitamin D intoxication
- Tumor lysis syndrome
- Laxative (Phospho-soda) abuse
- Rhabdomyolysis
- Hypoparathyroidism
- Pseudohypoparathyroidism
- Multiple myeloma

Treatment

- If greater than 4.5 mg/dL then:

- Treat the underlying cause
- Restrict calcium phosphate intake
- IV Normal Saline (if normal renal fx)
- Acetazolamide (500mg IV q6hr) - if normal renal function
- Phosphate Binder - Aluminum hydroxide (50-150mg/kg PO q4-6h) - limited effect
- Dialysis if refractory

HYPOPHOSPHATEMIA

- Phosphate required in function of all hematologic cells (RBCs, WBCs, platelets) and when low can cause:
  - Weakness
  - Circumoral and fingertip paresthesias
  - Decreased DTRs
  - Decreased Mental Status
  - Impaired myocardial function

Causes

- **Internal redistribution**
  - Refeeding of malnourished
  - DKA
  - Nonketotic hyperglycemia
  - Receiving hyperalimentation
  - Acute respiratory alkalosis
  - Hungry bone syndrome
- **Decreased intestinal absorption**
  - Inadequate intake
  - Antacids containing aluminum or magnesium
  - Steatorrhea and/or chronic diarrhea
- **Increased urinary excretion**
  - Vitamin D deficiency or resistance
  - Primary renal phosphate wasting (rare genetic disorders)
  - Multiple myeloma
  - Osmotic diuresis

- Proximally acting diuretics (e.g. acetazolamide and some thiazide diuretics)
- Acute volume expansion
- Intravenous iron administration
- Renal replacement therapy (dialysis)

Treatment

- **Serum phosphate 1mg/dl to 2mg/dl**
  - If able to take PO
    - Minimize or eliminate all dextrose-containing IV solutions
    - Aggressively treat acidosis
    - 1 tab K-phos neutral 250mg Q hour x 5 doses
    - Each tab contains phosphorus 8 mmol, Na 13 mEq, K1.1 mEq
    - Recheck serum phosphate after last dose, and repeat dosing if continues to be <2mg/dl
  - If NOT able to take PO
    - Minimize or eliminate all dextrose-containing IV solutions
    - Aggressively treat acidosis
    - Give 15 mmol of IV potassium phosphate over 2.5 hours (contains 22 mEq K)
    - Peripheral administration may cause burning at injection site
    - Consider central venous administration, if available
    - Repeat dosing regimen if serum phosphate remains <2mg/dl
- **Serum phosphate <1mg/dl**
  - Minimize or eliminate all dextrose-containing IV solutions
  - Aggressively treat any acidosis
  - Give 45 mmol of IV potassium phosphate over 7 hours (contains 66 mEq of K)
  - If patient can tolerate PO, ALSO follow steps 1 above
  - Recheck serum phosphate after infusion
    - Repeat IV administration if <1mg/dl
    - Consider oral administration if >1mg and <2mg/dl

HYPONATREMIA

- Defined as sodium concentration <135meq/L
- Patients often not symptomatic until <120meq/L, although this level varies by patients and may be higher if the change occurred abruptly
- Rapid correction (>10 meq/L/day), especially if chronic, can cause osmotic demyelination syndrome (central pontine myelinolysis)

Isotonic (pseudo) hyponatremia

- Defined as osmolarity > 275-295mmol/L. Often referred to as pseudo hyponatremia because the elevated lipids or proteins interfere with the laboratory sodium reading. The following are common causes:
- **Hyperlipidemia**
- **Hyperproteinemia**

Hypertonic Hyponatremia

- Defined as osmolarity > 295mmol/L with the following causes:
- **Hyperglycemia**
    - Sodium decreases by 2.4mEq/L for each 100mg/dL increase in glucose over 100mg/dL
- **Mannitol excess**

Hypotonic Hyponatremia causes by volume status

- Defined as an osmolarity < 275 mmol/L and categorized as **hypovolemic, hypervolemic or euvolemic**
- **Hypovolemic**
    - Renal Causes
        - Thiazide diuretic use
        - Na-wasting nephropathy (RTA, CRF)
        - Osmotic diuresis (glucose, urea)
        - Aldosterone deficiency
    - Extra-renal Causes
        - GI loss
        - 3rd space loss
        - Burns
        - Pancreatitis

- Peritonitis
- **Hypervolemic**
  - Urinary Na >20 indicates:
    - Renal losses
  - Urinary Na <20 indicates:
    - Nephrotic syndrome
    - Cirrhosis
    - CHF
- **Euvolemic**
  - SIADH
  - urine sodium is greater than 20-40 mEq/L
  - Pain, stress, nausea
  - Psychogenic polydipsia
  - Hypothyroidism
  - Drugs
  - NSAIDs, sulfonylureas, wellbutrin
  - H20 intoxication
  - Glucocorticoid deficiency

Treatment

- Since most patients are euvolemic (hypervolemic and hypovolemic are extremely rare), volume repletion is rarely needed and should be held until diagnosis of etiology is made.

Seizure Management

- **Adults:**
  - 3% hypertonic saline 150 mL bolus over 20 min
  - Check serum sodium concentration after 20 min
  - Repeat infusion of 150 ml 3% hypertonic saline for the next 20 min
  - Repeat twice or until a target of 5 mmol/l increase in serum sodium concentration is achieved
  - Each 100 mL will raise sodium by ~2 mmol/l
  - In general, 200-400 mL of 3% hypertonic saline is reasonable dose in most adult patients with severe symptomatic

hyponatremia, which may be given IV over 1-2 hr until resolution of seizures.

- **Pediatrics:**
    - 2 mL/kg of 3% over 10-60 minutes can be infused with a repeat of up to 3 times.

Calculating Sodium Replacement Therapy

- Max correction 10mEq/L in first 24hr (8 mmol/l during every 24 h thereafter), until a serum sodium concentration of 130 mmol/l is reached (lowers risk of osmotic demyelination syndrome)
- First: calculate total body water
    - **TBW(kg) = Wt(kg) x 0.6 = [Wt(lb) x 0.45] x 0.6 = Wt(lb) x 0.27**
- Second: calculate mEq deficit
    - **(Desired Na - Measured Na) ~ must be ≤ 10**
- Third: Calculate NS rate to be given over 24hr
    - **NS rate (cc/hr) = TBW x mEq deficit x 0.27**
    - **If using 3% sodium chloride (to avoid volume overload) divide above rate by 3.33**

HYPERNATREMIA

- High = >150meq/L and almost always due to decreased total body water

Causes

- **Water loss:**
    - Decreased Intake
    - Water loss > Na loss (vomiting/diarrhea, excessive sweating)
    - Dialysis
    - Osmotic diuresis
    - Central DI
    - Nephrogenic DI
    - Thyroidtoxicosis
- **Sodium gain:**
    - Increased intake (hypertonic fluid or or Sod. Bicarb infusion)
    - Renal Na retention (secondary to poor perfusion)

Treatment

- **Avoid lowering Na more than 10-15 mEq/L/day (~0.5-1.0 mEq/L/hr initially)**
- Can target a 0.5 mEq/hr correction with 1/2NS
- Central DI treat with DDAVP
- **Free water deficit = (0.6 x wt in kg) x [(serum Na/140) – 1]**

HYPOKALEMIA

- In extreme situations can cause weakness, and intermittent paralysis, and AV blocks or Vfib/Vtach

Causes

- Intracellular shifts
- Decreased intake
- Increased loss (GI or renal)

Repletion

- Every 10mEq KCl can increase serum K by ~0.1mEq/L
- Correct hypomagnesemia to assist with K repletion

HYPERKALEMIA

- Defined as >5.5 mEq/L
- Consider pseudohyperkalemia (e.g. from hemolysis)
- Potassium secretion is proportional to flow rate and sodium delivery through distal nephron
- Pseudohyperkalemia: hemolyzed specimen, prolonged tourniquet use prior to blood draw, thrombocytosis or leukocytosis
- **Redistribution (shift from intracellular to extracellular space):**
    - Acidemia (see DKA)
    - Cellular breakdown: see Rhabdomyolysis/Crush syndrome, electrical/thermal burn, hemolysis, see Tumor lysis syndrome
- **Increased total body potassium:**
    - Inadequate excretion: Acute/chronic renal failure, Addison's disease, type 4 RTA

- Drug-induced: potassium-sparing diuretic (spironolactone), angiotensin converting enzyme inhibitors (ACE-I), nonsteroidal anti-inflammatory drugs (NSAIDs)
- Excessive intake: diet, blood transfusion
- **Other causes: succinylcholine, digitalis, beta-blockers**

Stabilize cardiac membranes

- Indicated if there are any ECG changes or evidence of arrhythmias. Consider if K >7 mEq/L
- **Calcium gluconate: Give 10ml of a 10% solution over 10 mins**
    - Only 1/3 the calcium compared to calcium chloride
    - Can cause hypotension due to osmotic shift
- **Calcium chloride 1 gram IV**
    - Give over 1 - 2 minutes
    - Extravasation is bad: use a good IV
    - Usually given in code situations
    - Takes effect in 15-30 minutes
    - Duration of action: 30 - 60 minutes [2]
    - Use caution in patients taking Digoxin although risk of Stone heart may be unsubstantiated [3]
    - Do serial ECGs to track progress: may need to give multiple doses

Shift K+ intracellularly

- Intravenous insulin + dextrose
    - Give 10 units regular insulin intravenously with 25 to 50 grams (1 - 2 50 mL ampules) of 50% dextrose (D50)
    - May withhold dextrose if blood sugar >300mg/dl (>17 mmol/L)
    - Duration of effect: 4 - 6 hours
    - Consider mixing in 10 cc NS syringe to ensure small volume of 10 units insulin fully administered via IV
    - Insulin cleared renally, be careful about inducing hypoglycemia (ESRD patients).
    - In a small 2017 retrospective cohort study, researchers found that giving 5 units of insulin instead of 10 units reduced serum potassium to the same extent as 10 units, with a lower rate of hypoglycemia.

- **Nebulized albuterol 10 - 20mg**
    - Response is dose-dependent
    - Peak effect: 30 minutes
    - Duration of effect: 2 hours
- **Intravenous sodium bicarbonate 50ml of 8.4% solution (1 ampoule) given over 5 minutes**
    - Duration of effect: 1 - 2 hours
    - Generally not required, unless pH <7.1

Remove K+ from body

- Intravenous furosemide (Lasix) 40 - 80mg
- Sodium polystyrene sulfonate (Kayexalate): 30 gm oral or per rectum
- Sodium zirconium cyclosilicate
    - Potassium binder, similar to Kayexalate
- Intravenous normal saline solution for volume expansion if dehydrated, rhabdomyolysis, diabetic ketoacidosis or other acidosis
- Hydrocortisone if suspicious for adrenal insufficiency
- Definitive treatment is hemodialysis

Toxicology

TOXICITY BY PHARMACOLOGIC CLASS:

	Cholinergic	Anticholinergic	Sympathomimetic	Sympatholytic	Sedative/ Hypnotic
	Organophosphates	TCAs	Cocaine	Clonidine	ETOH
Temp	normal	increase	increased	normal/decreased	normal/ decreased
RR	Variable	decrease	Variable	normal/decreased	normal/ decreased
HR	Variable	increase	increased	normal/decreased	normal/ decreased
BP	increase	increase	increased	normal/decreased	normal/ decreased
LOC	Nl / Lethargic	Nl, agitated, psychotic, comatose	Nl, agitated, psychotic	Lethargic, or Comatose	Nl, Lethargic, or Comatose
Pupils	Variable	Mydriatic	Mydriatic	Nl / Miotic	n/a
Motor	Fasciculations, Flacid Paralysis	normal	Nl / Agitated	Nl	n/a
Skin	Sweating (sig)	Hot, dry	Sweating	Dry	n/a
Lungs	Bronchospasm / rhinorrhea	normal	Nl	Nl	n/a
Bowels	Hyperactive (SLUDGE)	decreased / Absent	normal	normal	normal

ALCOHOL WITHDRAWAL

- Withdrawal symptoms occur due to reduced GABA and increased NMDA receptors
- Tremulousness 6-12hrs after last drink
- Seizure occur 6-48hrs after last drink
- Delirium tremens 24hrs+ after last drink
- Treatment should favor maximal benzodiazepine dosing with redosing and doubling ever 15 minutes until symptoms resolve
  - Diazepam 10 mg IV every 15min with doubling
  - Lorazepam 2mg IV

- Barbiturates activate GABA channels via alternative pathway than benzos and are used for the benzodiazepine resistant withdrawal patient (Diazepam 200mg + or lorazepam 20mg+ without effect)
- Propofol sedation for those require intubation offers the best physiologic profile
- Chlordiazepoxide outpatient taper 50mg of chlordiazepoxide every 8 hours for two days, then decrease to 25mg every 8 hours for another two days followed by 25mg PRN as needed

ACETAMINOPHEN TOXICITY

Adult toxic dose

- 10 g or >200 mg/kg as single ingestion or over 24hr period **or**
- >6 g per day period for > 48hrs

Pediatric toxic dose

- >150 mg/kg per day for >48hrs
- 200 mg/kg in healthy children 1-6 years of age

150 Rule

- Toxic dose is 150 mg/kg
- Give NAC if level is >150 mcg/mL four hours post-ingestion
- Initial loading dose of NAC is 150 mg/kg IV (140 mg/kg PO)
- Acetaminophen (APAP) 4 hrs post-ingestion correlated to the Rumack-Matthew nomogram (can only be used for acute ingestions not chronic toxicity)
- Chronic ingestions with elevated LFTs, or an altered coagulation panel, or pH<7.3 and an acetaminophen level > 20mcg/mL should receive NAC therapy

NSAID TOXICITY

- Generally ingestions <100mg/kg are asymptomatic
- Ingestions > 400mg/kg can present with abdominal pain, hyperkalemia, renal insufficiency, metabolic acidosis, and in rare cases, shock.

SALICYLATE TOXICITY

- Salicylic acid is found in aspirin, oil of wintergreen, wart removers, maalox, alka-seltzer, muscle balms, and Pepto-Bismol

Mild toxicity (<150mg/kg)

- Tinnitus and nausea/vomiting

Moderate toxicity (150-300mg/kg)

- Hyperthermia and ataxia

Severe toxicity (>300mg/kg)

- Altered mental status, seizures, acute renal failure, and shock

Physiologic effects of toxicity

- Nausea/vomiting caused by chemoreceptor stimulation
- Respiratory alkalosis cause by activation of the respiratory center of the medulla
- Anion gap metabolic acidosis
- Hyperthermia from uncoupled oxidative phosphorylation
- As pH drops more ASA is uncharged and able to cross the blood brain barrier causing altered mental status
- Salicylates are directly toxic to brain tissue causing cerebral edema
- Pulmonary edema caused by increased pulmonary vascular permeability

TRICYCLIC ANTIDEPRESSANT TOXICITY

- >10mg/kg is life-threatening and causes:

Na Channel Blockade

- Negative inotropy, heart block, hypotension, ectopy

Anti-Histamine Effects

- Sedation, coma

Anti-Muscarinic Effects

- Mydriasis, dry skin, intestinal ileus, urinary retention, hyperthermia

α1 Receptor Blockade

- Sedation, orthostatic hypotension, miosis

- **Inhibition of amine reuptake**

- Sympathomimetic effects
- Myoclonus, hyperreflexia
- Rarely serotonin effects

SSRI TOXICITY

- Most serious adverse effect is potential to produce serotonin syndrome
  - **Myoclonus: most common finding**
  - **Agitated delirium**
  - **Autonomic instability (hyperthermia, tachycardia, hypertension, diaphoresis)**

Treatment:
  - Benzodiazepines to control agitation
  - Cyproheptadine (serotonin antagonist) if benzos are insufficient
  - Dexmedetomidine my assist for severe refractory cases
  - Aggressive cooling for hyperthermia

WHOLE BOWEL IRRIGATION

- Controversial therapy but may be useful for increasing gut transit of iron, lithium, or for body packers

ACTIVATED CHARCOAL

- 1g/kg (max 50g)
- Consider if toxic ingestion that occur within 1-2hr of presentation
- Does not bind with metals, hydrocarbons, caustics, or alcohols

COMMON ANTIDOTES AND POISON

Acetaminophen	N-Acetylcysteine
Aspirin	Sodium bicarb and/or dialysis
Organophosphates	Atropine, pralidoxime
Warfarin	Vitamin K, Prothombin Complex Concentrate or FFP
Digoxin	Digibind (Fab fragments)
Methanol/Ethylene glycol	Fomepizole
HFl acid	Topical calcium, magnesium
Isoniazid	Pyridoxine
Methanol	Fomepizole or ethanol, HD
TCAs	Sodium bicarb
Carbon monoxide	Oxygen and hyperbaric oxygen
Beta-blocker or calcium channel blocker overdose	Glucagon, high-dose insulin (intralipid therapy for extreme cases)
Iron	Deferoxamine
Cyanide	Hydroxocobalamin (historically: sodium nitrate, amyl nitrate, and sodium thiosulfate)

HEMODIALYSIS FOR TOXIC INGESTIONS

- Methanol or ethanol, salicylates, theophylline, lithium
- No effective for volumes that are lipophilic or with large volumes of distribution such as digoxin

ALCOHOLIC KETOACIDOSIS

- Seen in patients with recent history of binge drinking with little/no nutritional intake and therefore depleted glycogen stores with ketosis and hypo or eu-glycemia
- Characterized by high serum ketone levels and an elevated AG
- Acetoacetate is metabolized to acetone so elevated osmolal gap may also be seen
- Consider other causes of elevated AG, as well as co-ingestions (toxic alcohols, salicylates)
- Treatment is focused on dextrose repletion via IV fluids such as D5NS and electrolyte replacement
- Acidosis will quickly resolve after dextrose administration and patients can often be discharged once tolerating oral intake

WERNICKE-KORSAKOFF SYNDROME

- **Wernicke's Encephalopathy:** acute neurologic symptoms caused by thiamine deficiency
  - **Nystagmus/ophthalmoplegia**
  - **Incoordination/ataxia**
  - **Confusion/memory impairment**
- **Korsakoff's Psychosis:** chronic neurologic symptoms caused by thiamine deficiency

TOXIC ALCOHOL POISONING

Alcohol dehydrogenase metabolizes ethanol and toxic alcohols to their metabolites
- Is inhibited by fomepizole and ethanol

Ethylene Glycol Toxicity

- Metabolized by alcohol dehydrogenase to glycolic acid causes anion gap metabolic acidosis) and eventually oxalic acid
- Found in antifreeze, automobile coolants, de-icing agents, industrial solvents and hydraulic brake fluid.

Methanol Toxicity

- Metabolized to formaldehyde by alcohol dehydrogenase then formic acid (causes anion gap metabolic acidosis)

Isopropanol

- Primary ingredient in rubbing alcohol
- **Metabolized to acetone by alcohol dehydrogenase which causes a ketosis without an acidosis**

URINE DRUG SCREEN

Pertinent drugs not on a urine drug screen

- Fentanyl/Carfentil
- Methadone
- Synthetic marijuna
- Hallucinogens (LSD/MDM/Psilocybin)

Drug detection Interval after last use

- Amphetamines - 1-2 days
- Barbiturates - 2-4 days
- Benzodiazepines - 1-30days
- Cannabinoids - 1-3 days
- Cocaine - 2 days
- Opiates - 1-4 days
- Phencyclidine 4-7 days

MEDICATION ADVERSE EFFECTS

Aminoglycosides

- Ototoxicity
- Nephrotoxicity

Chloramphenicol

- Grey baby syndrome (cardiovascular depression)

Dapsone

- Prolonged use can cause methemoglobinemia
- Hemolysis if G6PD deficient

Ethambutol

- Optic neuritis
- Peripheral neuropathy

Isoniazid

- Seizures from GABA inhibition
- Treat with pyridoxine

Macrolide (azithromycin, clarithromycin, erythromycin)

- QT prolongation

Metronidazole

- Disulfiram-like reaction if taken with ethanol

Nitrofurantoin

- Hemolysis if G6PD deficient

Fluoroquinolones

- QT prolongation
- Tendinopathy (especially in pediatric patients)

Sulfonamides (TMP-SMX)

- Hemolysis if G6PD deficient
- Stevens-Johnson syndrome

Vancomycin

- Ototoxicity
- Nephrotoxicity
- "Red man" syndrome if infused quickly

Acyclovir

- Crystalluria

Nucleoside reverse transcription inhibitors

- Pancreatitis

Protease Inhibitors

- Dyslipidemia and Insulin-resistance during prolonged use

Haloperidol

- Dystonia
- Neuroleptic Malignant Syndrome (NMS)

Ondansetron

- QT prolongation

Metoclopramide

- QT prolongation
- Dystonia
- Akathisia

CARBON MONOXIDE TOXICITY

- Can coexist with cyanide toxicity
- Displaces oxygen from hemoglobin causing profound cellular hypoxia
- Pulse oximetry may read normal despite elevated carbon monoxide
- Half-Life
  - Room air: 5hrs
  - 100% O2: 1hr
  - HBO 2.5atm: 24min
- Normal carboxyhemoglobin <5% (smokers can be 8-10%)
- 10% COHb - confusion and agitation
- 20-30% COHb - nausea/vomiting, altered mental state
- 40-60% - unconscious
- >60% coma/death

- Three HBO treatments within 24hrs may reduce risk of cognitive sequelae 6 weeks and 12 months after CO poisoning (generally reserved for patients with 20% COHb and greater or if pregnant)
- Fetal Hb will bind CO to greatest degree

METHYLENE CHLORIDE

- Found in varnish and wood stain remover
- Can induce carbon monoxide toxicity

CLONIDINE TOXICITY

- Initial presentation manifests with hypotension and reflex tachycardia from alpha-1 agonism

DIGOXIN TOXICITY

- Digoxin Inhibits Na+/K+ ATPase in the myocardium causing increases in intracellular sodium levels which increases cardiac contractility
- Mortality is greatest in chronic ingestions due to the delay in diagnosis and increased rate of ventricular dysrhythmias
- Dysrhythmias occur from increased automaticity
    - PVCs (most common)
    - Bradycardia
    - SVT with AV block
    - Junctional escape
    - Atrial tachycardia or atrial fibrillation
    - Bidirectional V-tach

Digitalis Effect (seen at therapeutic levels or toxic levels)
- T wave changes (flattening or inversion)
- QT interval shortening
- **Scooped ST segments with depression in lateral leads**
- Increased U-wave amplitude

Symptoms
- Nausea/vomiting often the earliest manifestation of toxicity
- Confusion, delirium, Visual disturbances (yellow halos, scotomas)

- Hyperkalemia seen in acute poisoning
- Hypokalemia or hypomagnesemia can occur in chronic toxicity
- Treat with digoxin immune fab

CYANIDE TOXICITY

- Inhibits the electron transport chain preventing aerobic metabolism despite adequate oxygen saturation
- Should be suspected in anyone after smoke/fire exposure who has a lactic acidosis (anaerobic metabolism)
- **Presents with:**
    - CNS stimulation (Headache, anxiety, confusion)
    - Hypotension
    - Cherry-red color (rarely seen)
    - Lactic acidosis
- Classic smell is that of "bitter almonds"
- PO2 of venous blood approaches that of the arterial blood due to the aerobic metabolism inhabitation
- Serum cyanide levels have little utility unlike carbon monoxide level

Cyanokit (Hydroxocobalamin) - 1st line therapy

- 1st line therapy and should be given empirically if poisoning is suspected
- Directly binds cyanide forming cyanocobalamin which is readily excreted in the urine
- 70mg/kg IV over 15min (5g is standard adult dose)

Cyanide Antidote Package (Lilly kit) - 2nd line therapy

- A two drugs antidote (2 nitrites and a thiosulfate).
- The nitrites convert the iron in hemoglobin from the ferrous to the ferric form, creating methemoglobinemia.
- The thiosulfate is a sulfate donor, which allows the enzyme rhodanese to convert the cyanide to a form that can be renally excreted.
- Consider using only Na thiosulfate (no nitrites) in cases where concern for CO poisoning since nitrate administration will severely decrease oxygen carrying capacity

BETA-BLOCKER OR CALCIUM CHANNEL TOXICITY

- Beta blocker toxicity often manifests with hypoglycemia as compared to calcium channel blocker toxicity
- Treatment options should primarily focus on supportive care to avoid cardiovascular collapse, however high-dose insulin or intravenous lipid emulsion are emerging therapies

Glucagon

- 5mg IV bolus q10min x 2
- Will often cause severe nausea/vomiting, give Zofran prior

Vasopressor support

- Norepinephrine initiate at 2mcg/min, with goal MAP 65mmHg

High-dose insulin and glucose

- Insulin provides positive inotropic effect by encouraging the heart to use glucose metabolism as their primary energy source).
- Insulin at 1 unit/kg/hr with glucose checks every 15 minutes and dextrose infusions
- Potassium checks every hour with continuous potassium repletion (oral and peripheral)

Intravenous lipid emulsion

- 1.5mL/kg bolus of 20% lipid followed by 0.25mL/kg/minute

ANTI-CHOLINERGIC CRISIS

Medications causes

- Atropine
- Lomotil
- Antihistamines
- Tricyclic antidepressant (TCA) toxicity
- SSRIs
- Antipsychotics
- Muscle relaxants
- Anti-Parkinsonians

• Plants (Jimson weed, Amanita mushroom)

Symptoms

- Dry as a bone: anhydrosis
- Hot as a hare: hyperthermia
- Red as a beet: cutaneous vasodilation
- Blind as a bat: nonreactive mydriasis
- Mad as a hatter: delirium
- Full as a flask: urinary retention
- Tachycardia (HR 120-160) and decreased/absent bowel sounds

Treatment

- Benzodiazepines for seizures
- Sodium bicarbonate for QRS prolongation
- Cholinesterase inhibition (physostigmine) should only be given in coordination with a toxicologist due to the risk of cholinergic crisis

LOCAL ANESTHETICS

- Lidocaine without epinephrine: 4 mg/kg max dose
- Lidocaine with epinephrine: 7 mg/kg max dose
- Treatment anesthetic toxicity with intralipid infusion

"Amides" vs "Esters"

- Amides have 2 "i's in the name (e.g. lidocaine, bupivacaine)
- Esters have 1 "i" (e.g. procainamide and cocaine)
- Generally patients are only allergic to one class

Cetacaine and benzocaine spray

- **In high doses may produce methemoglobinemia**
- Treatment with methylene blue

CROTALIDAE ENVENOMATION

- Rattlesnakes (copperhead and cottonmouth)
- Thrombin-like venom causing cytotoxicity

- Anti-venom (crofab) for severe rapidly expanding bites or if compartment syndrome develops

ELAPIDAE ENVENOMATION

- Coral snakes
- Venom causes neurotoxic and respiratory depression
- Anti-venom is less commonly available and often acquired from zoos
- The following acronym is not valid in Latin American or South America
- **Red on yellow, kill a fellow (for deadlier coral snakes)**
- **Red on black, venom lack (king cobras)**

GAMMA-HYDROXYBUTYRIC ACID (GHB)

- Acute toxicity causes immediate sedation with a wakeup with a few hours
- Chronic use can lead to withdrawal symptoms similar to alcohol withdrawal

PCP AND KETAMINE

- Patients have a characteristic rotatory nystagmus

NEUROLEPTIC MALIGNANT SYNDROME (NMS)

- **Tetrad of:**
  - **Altered mental status**
  - **Muscular Rigidity**
  - **Hyperthermia >38C**
  - **Autonomic Instability**
- Majority of deaths occur from complications of muscle rigidity
- Can occur with single dose, increasing dose, or same dose as usual
- Most often seen with "typical" high potency antipsychotics (haldol)

DIFFERENTIATING NMS FROM OTHER CONDITIONS

Serotonin Syndrome

- More likely to have hyperreflexia and myoclonus
- Rigidity and hyperthermia, if present, is less severe than in NMS

Malignant Hyperthermia

- Distinguish by clinical setting (use of inhalational anesthetics or sux)
- Hyperthermia, muscle rigidity, and dysautonomia is similar to NMS though more fulminant

Anticholinergic Toxicity

- Diaphoresis, rigidity, elevated CK are absent
- Flushing, mydriasis and bladder distention

Sympathomimetics

- Rigidity does not occur

MALIGNANT HYPOTHERMIA

- Inherited disorder of skeletal muscles triggered most often by anesthesia inhalation agents, succinylcholine, heat or exercise

CAUSTIC INGESTIONS

- Solid chemical exposure can cause a more proximal injury (oropharynx and proximal esophagus).
- Liquids cause more distal injury (gastric and intestinal).
- Substances that cause injury to organic tissues upon contact
- **Acid: pH < 3**
  Damages tissues with coagulative necrosis.
- **Base (Alkali): pH > 11**
  Damages tissues with liquefactive necrosis - achieves deeper penetration.
- Never neutralize the acid or base (releases heat and other chemical byproducts).
- Never induce emesis.

HYDROFLUORIC ACID (HF)

- Strong acid found in scenarios that involve etching, metal and rust cleaners:
- The fluoride ion reacts with calcium and magnesium to deplete local and systemic stores.
- Hypocalcemia and hyperkalemia from tissue breakdown and acidosis lead to death by cardiac arrest.
- Delayed and prolonged exposure (low concentration HF) causes greatest harm due to greatest duration of calcium sequestration and tissue damage.
- Calcium gluconate gel - Applied to the exposed area can bind free fluoride ions and prevent further skin damage. Secondary treatment can include subcutaneous 5-10% calcium gluconate for refractory pain. Systemic therapy involves IV calcium gluconate.

WHITE PHOSPHORUS

- Common in methamphetamine labs - causes nausea and vomiting and is highly flammable.
- Garlic odor
- Treatment: removal from the environment and decontamination

Trauma

CT SCAN MISSED INJURIES

- Diaphragm (mostly in penetrating trauma)
- Hollow viscus (bowel)

SEAT BELT SIGN

- Increases the risk of a hollow viscus injury and spinal fracture

FAST EXAM LIMITATIONS

- Cannot detect retroperitoneal blood
- Requires 250-500mL of blood for positive visualization

EMERGENT OR ADMISSION

- Eviscerated abdominal contents
- Peritonitis in blunt or penetrating trauma
- Positive FAST exam in an unstable patient

HARD SIGNS OF ARTERIAL INJURY

- Visible arterial bleeding
- Rapidly expanding hematoma (or pulsatile hematoma)
- Absent pulses
- Thrill or brui
- Distal ischemia

SOFT SIGNS OF ARTERIAL INJURY

- Non-expanding hematoma
- Injury in proximity to an artery
- Transient or unexplained hypotension
- Nerve injury

- <0.5 - arterial injury until proven otherwise
- 0.5-0.9 - probable arterial injury
- >0.9 - unlikely an arterial injury

RETROPERITONEAL TRAUMA

- CT is best diagnostic test
- Aorta, pancreas, kidney, inferior vena cava, duodenum, ascending and descending colon

INJURY GRADES (1-5)

- Grade 1 - least severe with a small laceration (requires observation)
- Grade 5 - organ destruction requiring operative bleeding control

TRAUMATIC CARDIAC TAMPONADE

- May manifest with hypotension, distant heart sounds, and JVD (beck's triad)
- Treat with thoracotomy or pericardiocentesis
- Survival is unlikely, especially with blunt trauma

LIMB AND DIGIT AMPUTATIONS

- Wrap the amputated limb or digit in saline soaked gauze
- Place gauze in watertight container
- Place container in an ice water bath
- Ensure ice never touches the limb or digit
- Reimplantation criteria
    - Pediatric patient
    - Thumb amputations
    - Singular clean severed digit
    - Multiple non macerated sequential digits
    - Entire hand or forearm amputation

HUMAN AND ANIMAL BITES

- Polymicrobial (Staph Strep) Plus
    - Humans: Eikenella
    - Dogs: Capnocytophagia
    - Cats: Pasteurella
- Generally clindamycin or amoxicillin/clavulanate covers all pertinent organisms

COMPARTMENT SYNDROME

- Pain out of proportion to exam in the setting of a tight extremity compartment (5 Ps) with a delta pressure or absolute pressure abnormality
    - Pain out of proportion
    - Paresthesia
    - Pallor
    - Paresis
    - Pulse deficit
- **Delta pressure = Diastolic BP - compartment pressure**
    - **Abnormal if < 30 mmHg**
- **Absolute Pressure > 30 mmHg**

CLAVICLE FRACTURES

- Majority are middle 1/3
- Only require emergent orthopedic consult if severely displaced and/or skin tenting

RIB FACTURES

- Flail chest: segmental fractures in 3 or more adjacent ribs
- Renal lacerations or other intraabdominal injuries can occur with low rib fractures

STERNAL FRACTURES

- Can be associated with aortic injuries or cardiac contusions

CARDIAC CONTUSIONS

- Most commonly injury the right ventricle (most anterior structure)
- Present with arrhythmia and/or troponin elevation
- Require supportive care

PULMONARY CONTUSIONS

- Direct injury to lung resulting in hemorrhage and edema
- Visible > 6 hours post injury as patchy infiltrates
- Patients with >25% of lung involvement frequently require ventilatory assistance (CPAP/BIPAP)

THORACOTOMY

- Consider if originally signs of life and then an arrest
- Although chance of survival is low, it is best if performed within 10-15 min of witnessed arrest

TENSION PNEUMOTHORAX

- JVD, tachycardia, hypotension, tracheal deviation due to increased intrathoracic pressure
- Require immediate needle decompression or chest tube

TRAUMATIC AORTIC DISSECTION

- Often distal to left subclavian artery at ligamentum arteriosum
- Chest Xray may have mediastinal widening or tracheal/esophageal deviation
- CTA of the chest is ideal for diagnosis

CORNEAL INJURIES

- Abrasions - will demonstrate fluorescence uptake and require topical antibiotics (cessation of contact lenses until healed)
- Alkaline injuries to cornea can occur from airbag inflation chemicals
- Globe lacerations - may demonstrate Seidel's sign (waterfall after fluorescence)

LATERAL CANTHOTOMY

- Suspected acute orbital compartment syndrome (OCS), plus one or more of the following:
    - Decreased visual acuity
    - IOP >40 **or** marked difference in globe compressibility by palpation
    - Proptosis

TRAUMATIC IRITIS

- Blunt trauma causes a contusion and spasm of the ciliary body and iris
- Direct and consensual photophobia
- Treat with a long acting cycloplegic (homatropine) to prevent ciliary spasm

LE FORT FRACTURE

- Mid-face fracture involving the maxilla and surrounding facial structures

Le Fort I

- Stable fracture above the dental arch
- Only hard palate and teeth move

Le Fort II

- Often unstable fracture through pyramidal fracture through central maxilla and hard palate
- Movement of hard palate and nose occurs

Le Fort III

- Craniofacial dysfunction
- Unstable fracture through frontozygomatic sutures, orbit, nose, and ethmoids
- Entire face shifts with globes held in place only by optic nerve

Le Fort IV

- Le Fort III plus involvement of frontal bone (unstable)

GLOBE RUPTURE

Clinical signs:

- Afferent pupillary defect (fail swinging flashlight test)
- Teardrop pupil
- Seidel sign
- Uveal prolapse (brown/black discoloration at site where uvea or iris is herniating)
- Bullous subconjunctival hemorrhage

NASAL SEPTAL HEMATOMA

- Must be drained otherwise septal necrosis can occur

DENTAL FRACTURE

- Ellis 1: through enamel
- Ellis 2: through dentin (yellow middle layer)
  - Cover with calcium hydroxide paste over exposed dentin
- Ellis 3: exposed pulp (blood or pink color)
  - Cover area with moist gauze with emergent dental followup due to infection risk

INTRACRANIAL HEMORRHAGE

- Cerebral Perfusion Pressure = Mean Arterial Pressure - Intracranial Pressure
- If lesion causes increase in intracranial pressure, patients may manifest a Cushing's response:
  - Hypertension
  - Bradycardia
  - Bradypnea
- In addition to neurosurgical consultation, management should focus on seizure prophylaxis, avoidance of hypotension, and correction of any coagulopathies
- Head of bed elevation to 30 degrees to decrease intracranial pressure

- Avoid hypoventilation (in intubated patients) due to unpredictability of effects and risk of hypocapnea causing vasoconstriction reducing blood flow

Subarachnoid Hemorrhage
- CTA to rule out aneurysmal rupture

Epidural Hematoma
- High associated with skull fractures and additional cerebral injuries

Subdural Hematoma
- Sudden acceleration-deceleration of the brain with resultant shearing of the bridging veins

TBI BY GCS

- Severe (GCS <8)
- Moderate (GCS 9-13)
- Mild (GCS 14-15)
- Patients with TBI have increased mortality and morbidity with prehospital hypotension (SBP < 90 mmHg).

DIFFUSE AXONAL INJURY

- Shows loss of grey-white differentiation on CT scan and often portends poor neurologic recovery

BASILAR SKULL FRACTURE SIGNS

- Battle's sign (mastoid ecchymosis)
- Raccoon's eyes (periorbital ecchymosis)
- Hemotympanum
- CSF rhinorrhea

ZONES OF THE NECK

- I - Sternal notch to cricoid cartilage
- II - Cricoid cartilage to angle of mandible

- III - Angle of mandible to base of skull
- Zone II injuries should have surgical exploration while I and III can have imaging first to rule out aero-digestive injuries
- Violation of the platysma should prompt imaging or surgical exploration

UNSTABLE CERVICAL SPINE FRACTURES

- Jefferson's fracture
    - C1 burst fracture due to axial load
- Bilateral Cervical facet dislocation
    - Hyperflexion
- Odontoid fracture, type II or III
- Atlante-Occipital dissociation
- Hangman's fracture
    - Hyperextension with bilateral C2 pedicle fractures
- Flexion teardrop
    - Often at C5-C6
- **Mnemonic: "Jefferson Bit Off A Hangman's Thumb"**

PENILE FRACTURE

- Tunica albuginea of one or both corpus cavernosa ruptures due to trauma to erect penis
- Emergent urologic repair
- Retrograde urethrogram can rule out associated urethral injury

URETHRAL INJURY

- Can occur with lower pelvic trauma
- Retrograde urethrogram to diagnose

BLADDER INJURY

- Presents with frank hematuria also associated with pelvic trauma
- Retrograde cystogram to diagnose

MASSIVE TRANSFUSION (MTP)

- Transfusion of >10 units of PRBCs
- 1:1:1 ratio of FFP:Platelet:PRBCs
- Some MTP protocols also include Tranexamic acid (TXA) to be administered 3 hours after injury

LETHAL TRIAD OF TRAUMA

- Hypothermia
- Coagulopathy
- Acidosis

NEUROGENIC SHOCK

- Injury to cervical or thoracic vertebrae causes peripheral sympathetic denervation
  - Above T1: full sympathetic denervation
  - T1-L3: Partial sympathetic denervation
  - Below L4: no sympathetic denervation

SPINAL SHOCK

- Transient stunning of the cord with global loss of function (unlike neurogenic shock) with temporary loss of spinal cord function below complete or incomplete spinal cord injury
- Bulbocavernosus reflex (S2-S4) is among the first to return as spinal shock resolves

BURNS

- Parkland Formula - 4 mL x patient weight (kg) x %TBSA = 24-hour fluid requirement.
- 50% given in first 8 hrs.
- For children <30 kg use 3 mL x patient weight (kg).
- Children require an additional 1mL/kg/hr added in maintenance fluids.

BODY SURFACE ESTIMATION CHART

	Adult	Child
Anterior Head	4.5%	9%
Posterior Head	4.5%	9%
Entire head is 9% for adults but 18% for children.		
Anterior Torso	18%	18%
Posterior Torso	18%	18%
Anterior leg (per leg)	9%	6.75%
Posterior leg (per leg)	9%	6.75%
Anterior arm (per arm)	4.5%	4.5
Posterior arm (per arm)	4.5%	4.5
Entire arm for adults and children is 9%.		
Perineum	1%	1
Rule of 9s only includes partial thickness and greater.		

BURN CLASSIFICATION BY DEPTH

Degree	Classification	Appearance	Sensation
1st	**Superficial**	Red **blanching** skin (sunburn)	Painful
2nd	**Superficial partial thickness**	**Blistering** with red blanching skin	Painful to air
	Deep partial thickness	Blisters with **unroofing** and wet mixed white/red tissue - minimal to no blanching	Only pressure sensation
3rd	**Full thickness**	Waxy to leathery **white** and gray or charred - non- blanching	Superficially **insensate** and minimal sensation to deep pressure

BURNS REQUIRING BURN CENTER CARE

- Partial thickness burns greater than 10% TBSA.
- Burns that involve the face, hands, feet, genitalia, perineum or major joints.
- Full thickness burns in any age group.
- Electrical burns, including lightning injury.
- Chemical burns.
- Inhalation injury.
- Burn injury in a patient with preexisting medical disorders.
- Any patient with burns and concomitant trauma.
- Burned children in hospitals without qualified personnel and equipment.
- Burn injury in patients who will require social, emotional or rehabilitative intervention.

www.ingramcontent.com/pod-product-compliance
Lightning Source LLC
Chambersburg PA
CBHW042146220326
41599CB00003BB/9